Problems
in
Peripheral
Vascular Disease

Problems in Practice Series

Problems in Practice Series

Series Editors : J.Fry K.G.D.Williams M.Lancaster-Smith

Problems in Peripheral Vascular Disease

P.E.A.Savage

MS,FRCS

Consultant General and Vascular Surgeon
Queen Mary's Hospital,Sidcup,Kent

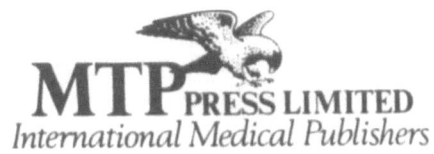

MTP PRESS LIMITED
International Medical Publishers

To

A.L.S.

Published by
MTP Press Limited
Falcon House
Lancaster, England

Copyright © 1983 P.E.A. Savage
Softcover reprint of the hardcover 1st edition 1983
First published 1983

British Library Cataloguing in Publication Data

Savage, Peter E.A.
   Problems in peripheral vascular disease
   —(Problems in practice)
   1. Peripheral vascular diseases 2. Ischaemia
   I. Title   II. Series
   616.1'31   RC694

ISBN-13: 978-94-011-6650-8   e-ISBN-13: 978-94-011-6648-5
DOI: 10.1007/978-94-011-6648-5

Butler & Tanner Ltd, Frome and London

Contents

Preface

In writing this short monograph on 'Problems in Peripheral Vascular Disease', I have tried to steer a course between a simplistic dogmatic approach more appropriate to an undergraduate text, and a detailed specialist treatise of interest only to vascular surgeons.

Although arterial surgery has been performed for centuries, the main indications in the past were to deal with the effects of trauma and aneurysm formation. The development of arteriography and the ability to see arterial blocks and stenoses allowed surgeons to carry out increasingly sophisticated operations for an enlarging range of pathological conditions. Even today, arterial surgery continues to develop, and although we are often dealing with the 'surgery of ruins', a successful outcome is just as rewarding for surgeon and patient alike.

In this book I have also included a discussion on venous problems including a note about recent developments in direct surgery of the deep veins of the lower limb which could be a rewarding field of endeavour for the vascular surgeon.

The original descriptions by Buerger and Raynaud are taken from 'Classic Descriptions of Disease' by Ralph H. Major. While reviewing my own surgical practice, I have had the pleasure of reading once again the publications of H.H.G. Eastcott (arterial surgery), J.T. Hobbs (varicose veins), G.L. Hill (Buerger's disease), Adrian Marston (intestinal ischaemia), Martin Birnstingl (vasospastic disorders) and C.H. Hawkes (lumbar canal stenosis).

To my registrar, Mr F. Massouh FRCS, I extend my thanks for the trouble he has taken in reading the draft manuscript and for making many valuable suggestions. My secretary, Mrs Sharon Hartman, has typed the manuscript with her usual patience and skill.

P.E.A. Savage
Sidcup, 1982

Series Foreword

This series of books is designed to help general practitioners. So are other books. What is unusual in this instance is their collective authorship; they are written by specialists working at district general hospitals. The writers derive their own experience from a range of cases less highly selected than those on which textbooks are traditionally based. They are also in a good position to pick out topics which they see creating difficulties for the practitioners of their district, whose personal capacities are familiar to them; and to concentrate on contexts where mistakes are most likely to occur. They are all well-accustomed to working in consultation.

All the authors write from hospital experience and from the viewpoint of their specialty. There are, therefore, matters important to family practice which should be sought not within this series, but elsewhere. Within the series much practical and useful advice is to be found with which the general practitioner can compare his existing performance and build in new ideas and improved techniques.

These books are attractively produced and I recommend them.

J.P. Horder CBE
Past President, The Royal College
of General Practitioners

9

1 Arterial occlusive disease

Presentation – Examination and risk factors – Investigations – Vasoactive drugs – Surgical treatment

The clinical features of arterial insufficiency in the lower limb are reflected by the relative needs of various tissues for oxygen and nourishment. Exercising muscle, being the most active metabolic tissue in a limb, registers its relative anoxia by stimulating pain receptors. This pain is brought on by exercise and relieved by rest. As the degree of ischaemia increases, the claudication distance becomes shorter until the patient suffers from continuous pain at rest. Progressive arterial insufficiency eventually leads to deterioration in skin nutrition with ulceration. The death of skin and deeper structures in the foot and leg is followed by infection and gangrene.

Presentation

Presenting complaint   A patient may consult his family doctor with three main peripheral vascular problems: an acute arterial occlusion (Chapter 5), a chronic arterial occlusion which has progressed to the stage at which viability of the limb is precarious (Chapter 3) and a chronic vascular insufficiency causing intermittent claudication.

Intermittent claudication   Although there are a number of causes for pain in the lower limb, pain in a muscle group brought on by exercise and completely relieved by rest is the classical presentation of intermittent claudication. Claudication may affect the muscles of the

11

foot, calf, thigh or buttock. The site of pain may be constant or the patient my find that over a period of time the muscle groups affected change, with more than one group becoming involved. The rate of change in the claudication distance is also important, and claudicants should be kept under review for at least 6 months provided that their symptoms are not obviously becoming disabling.

Anatomy of arterial blood supply

Knowledge of the arterial supply to the muscles of the lower limb allows the site of occlusion or stenosis to be localized. Thus the muscles of the foot are supplied by the branches of the plantar arch, the muscles of the calf by branches of the popliteal artery (anterior and posterior tibial arteries and peroneal artery), while the thigh muscles are supplied by the profunda femoris artery (the superficial femoral artery has no significant muscular branches) and the buttock muscles by branches of the internal iliac artery.

Examination and risk factors

Inspection

Clinical examination of both limbs allows a comparison to be made between the appearance, colour and temperature of both legs. The femoral, popliteal, dorsalis pedis and posterior tibial pulses are palpated and the stethoscope is applied to the femoral and iliac vessels to detect any bruit associated with an arterial stenosis. Evidence of subclavian or carotid artery stenosis or occlusion is sought by palpation and auscultation, and an abdominal aortic aneurysm excluded by examining the abdomen.

Palpation
Auscultation

Elevation and exercise test

A simple test of arterial blood supply is to ask the recumbent patient to raise both legs in the air, supporting them with his hands placed behind the thighs. In this position the feet are plantar- and dorsiflexed briskly by the patient to exercise the calf muscles while the doctor watches for any change in colour of the soles of the feet. When the patient complains of claudication, he is asked to sit up with the legs hanging down while the rate of venous filling of the foot veins is noted, comparing one side with the other. The degree in delay in venous filling and appearance of a postexercise capillary flush is an indication of the degree of arterial occlusion to the lower limb.

The assessment of symptomatic arterio-occlusive disease involves more than an analysis of the pathophysiology of the presenting symptoms. Patients are invariably heavy smokers, often overweight with other manifestations of atherosclerosis.

Many have evidence of ischaemic heart disease and some have already had a stroke.

Natural history of claudication

Risk factors

Intermittent claudication as a symptom on its own usually follows a benign course in that 60–70% of patients, when followed over a 5 year period, either remain unchanged or improve. Less than 5% require amputation within 5 years of presentation. Hypertension and diabetes, either unrecognized or under treatment, are frequently associated problems. Vascular reconstructive surgery is not to be lightly undertaken and these patients need a full assessment and appreciation of all the risk factors involved before surgery is advised.

Hypertension

Hypertension has long been recognized as a dangerous condition. Reduction of blood pressure to acceptable levels reduces the incidence of cerebrovascular accidents by 31% and of myocardial infarction by 21%. The features of coronary artery disease may be recognized on the electrocardiogram of 25% of all claudicants, and 20–30% of patients presenting with peripheral vascular disease are dead within 5 years, usually of a heart attack or stroke.

Myocardial ischaemia

Myocardial infarction

Patients who have had a myocardial infarction within the previous 3 months have a 36% risk of a further infarction while undergoing surgery; this risk falls to 7% for longer intervals.

Angina pectoris

Those with angina inadequately controlled by optimal medical treatment require cardiological assessment including coronary angiography to determine whether they should have a coronary artery bypass graft before embarking on a peripheral vascular reconstruction. Coronary artery bypass grafting (CABG) has an operative mortality of less than 1% and is now an established surgical procedure of proven value. While it is effective in relieving angina, its influence on long-term prognosis is still being evaluated.

CABG

Cigarette smoking

The medical treatment of a number of specific conditions is detailed in later chapters, but all patients with peripheral vascular disease are advised to stop smoking completely and never to start again. There is now considerable evidence that those patients with peripheral vascular disease who reduce or stop smoking have a much improved prognosis; in one series 11% of those claudicants who continued smoking came to amputation while those who stopped smoking kept both limbs intact. There is also good evidence of a higher graft failure rate in smokers than non-smokers. Some vascular surgeons now refuse elective arterial reconstruction to any patient who has not stopped smoking.

13

Hyperlipi-
daemia

Hyperlipidaemia is known to be a risk factor in the development of atherosclerosis and a serum cholesterol greater than
7.7 mmol/l has been shown to be of significance. A recent study
has suggested that it is possible to reduce the rate of atheroma
deposition in patients receiving lipid-lowering therapy by diet
and drugs.

Exercise

Regular exercise is an important factor in the management
of patients with intermittent claudication. Until the cause of
their symptoms is explained to them, many patients either try to
walk through the pain barrier, or stop walking altogether. By
understanding the importance of graduated exercises, the
patient is able to encourage collateral vessels to develop and
thus improve the blood supply to claudicating muscles.

Investigations

Haemoglobin

Investigations include an estimation of the haemoglobin to
exclude anaemia and polycythaemia, both of which will need
investigation and treatment. Diabetes mellitus is excluded by

Urinalysis

urinalysis, but the presence of sugar requires a random blood
sugar estimation and a glucose tolerance test. Syphilitic
arteritis is very rare in the United Kingdom but a suspicious

Serology
Fasting lipids

doctor will exclude it by serological tests. Fasting lipids indicate
whether any abnormality of fat metabolism requires correction

Chest X-ray
ECG Lung
function test

by diet, drugs or a combination of both. Cardiopulmonary status
is evaluated with the aid of a chest X-ray, electrocardiogram and
lung function tests.

Doppler ultra-
sound

One of the most useful techniques of investigating vascular
problems, both arterial and venous, is the Doppler ultrasound.
It will be recalled that the Doppler effect describes the change in
frequency of light or sound when an object moves away from, or
towards the observer. This principle is now used to receive an
audible signal from the movement of blood in a vessel. A high
frequency sound is emitted from a crystal in a probe placed over
the vessel being examined. The sound is transmitted through the
skin for a variable distance into the tissue where it is reflected back from a moving column of blood and received by
another crystal in the same probe. The difference in frequency
between the transmitted and received signal is converted into an
electric current which may output either as an audible sound or
as a waveform on a paper trace. By inflating a sphygmomano-
meter cuff around the lower calf, and listening with the Doppler
probe over the posterior tibial or dorsalis pedis arteries, the

systolic pressure at which the signal disappears can be recorded. The ratio of the ankle systolic pressure to the brachial systolic pressure is known as the pressure index, and in normal individuals is greater than 1.0. A pressure index of 0.5 or less is found in patients with calf claudication, and those with rest pain have an index less than 0.25.

Ankle pulses are often difficult to feel, and a simple Doppler probe is an invaluable diagnostic aid which should have a greater application in general practice.

Angiography   Although other non-invasive methods of imaging the arterial tree exist, no technique has yet replaced angiography. Radio-opaque contrast material may be introduced into an artery either by direct needle puncture of the vessel or by the Seldinger technique. Seldinger described a method of introducing a flexible guide wire through a needle inserted into an artery. After withdrawal of the needle, a flexible arterial catheter is passed over the guide wire which is withdrawn. The catheter may then be advanced in various directions so that selective angiograms of specific vessels can be obtained. Many angiograms are performed under a local anaesthetic but others, including lumbar arteriograms, are carried out with the patient anaesthetized. Like all invasive techniques, angiography has its complications, but these are infrequent when performed by a skilled, experienced radiologist.

Not every patient with peripheral vascular disease needs an arteriogram. The diagnosis of arterial occlusion or stenosis can usually be made on clinical assessment alone. Arteriography is necessary however, to provide information essential to plan a reconstructive vascular procedure. Three separate pieces of information are required, the site and extent of the occlusion or stenosis, the absence of any proximal obstruction to inflow, and the presence of an adequate outflow or run-off. Without a good inflow and a good run-off, even the most immaculate reconstruction is doomed to early failure.

Vasoactive drugs

To date, there is no evidence that antilipaemic drugs, anticoagulants, vasodilators or rheological agents confer any benefit to the patient with lower limb ischaemia. While antiplatelet drugs and prostaglandins may prevent further progression of atherosclerosis, convincing evidence has not yet been published. Naftidrofuryl and suloctidil may relieve pain of intermittent claudication, the former by its effect on improving ischaemic tissue's metabolic efficiency.

Surgical treatment

Vascular surgery for arterio-occlusive disease is the surgery of ruins. The surgeon is seldom able to say that he has cured the condition, and in the majority of cases the procedure has been essentially palliative. The indication for surgery depends on a balanced assessment of the severity of the symptoms, the interpretation of relevant angiograms, an appreciation of the likely result of surgery, and a knowledge of the operating surgeon's skills.

Assessment

Technique

The actual technique of vascular reconstruction is not particularly difficult, but greater care and precision are required as the diameter of the vessel being reconstructed gets smaller. Incisions in arteries are either longitudinal or transverse, and are closed with an over-and-over continuous suture of nonabsorbable material. In medium-size and small arteries, the closure of a longitudinal arteriotomy usually causes an unacceptable narrowing of the vessel. This is overcome by performing a patch angioplasty – a patch of vein or synthetic material being sutured to the cut edges of the arterial wall in order to widen the lumen.

Patch angioplasty

Thromboendarterectomy

Atheromatous plaques of limited length are removed by the technique of thromboendarterectomy (disobliteration, rebore). The artery is opened and a plane of cleavage developed between the layers of the media in which the atheroma is deposited. The adventitia of the arterial wall is its strongest layer, and provided this is kept intact together with a thin layer of media, the vessel wall is not significantly weakened. Although loose flaps attached to the wall of the artery above the endarterectomy site cause no concern, they become of crucial importance below as the force of the bloodstream can either lead to a dissection of the vessel wall, or the flap can swing across the lumen. In both events the outcome is the same, blood flow is impeded, thrombosis supervenes, and the reconstruction fails within a few hours.

Grafts

Longer stenoses or occlusions are dealt with by a grafting procedure. The graft may be (1) placed *in situ*, replacing the diseased vessel, (2) placed around the diseased segment as a bypass or (3) inserted in an extra-anatomic site such as an axillo-femoral or femorofemoral crossover graft.

Above the inguinal ligament in the aortoiliac segment where vessels are of large calibre and blood flow is brisk, synthetic grafts such as Dacron are successful. Below the inguinal ligament in the femoropopliteal segment with its smaller calibre and reduced blood flow, the best graft material is the patient's own reversed saphenous vein. On occasions this vein has already been stripped out, or is otherwise unsuitable. In this situation, polytetrafluoroethylene (PTFE Goretex) or human umbilical vein (Dardik) grafts may be used. Both these materials can be placed across the knee joint without kinking on knee-flexion and long-term patency rates are good.

PTFE
Umbilical
vein

Vascular surgery is an exacting and time-consuming specialty. A reconstructive operation may take 3-4 hours or longer and at the end of this, if a completion arteriogram is at all unsatisfactory, one or more anastomoses have to be repeated.

The surgical treatment of intermittent claudication

Assessment – Aortoiliac reconstruction – Femoropopliteal reconstruction

The aim of reconstructive surgery for intermittent claudication is to relieve the patient's symptoms with the minimum morbidity and no mortality. Surgical techniques are designed either to remove the atheromatous plaque and associated thrombus which is narrowing or blocking a major artery, or to bypass the diseased segment either with the patient's own saphenous vein or with a graft made of synthetic material. Dilatation of narrowed segments using a balloon catheter has a certain popularity with interventional radiologists but its role in the management of intermittent claudication has yet to be clearly defined.

Assessment

Degree of disability
The assessment of the patient's degree of disability is the crucial aspect of preoperative management. Disabling claudication does not lend itself to accurate definition. What may be an intolerable limitation on an active man in his 50s may be perfectly acceptable to someone 10 years older. As each patient's lifestyle is different, we should inquire carefully whether claudication is interfering with the ability to carry on normal work, or prevents enjoyment of reasonable leisure activities.

Pros and cons
Against any possible benefit to the patient from relief of his claudication must be weighed the disadvantages. Peripheral

19

vascular surgery is a time-consuming and exacting art. To the general risks of any major operation we have to add the risks of making the condition worse, the patient leaving hospital with no improvement in his claudication distance, or the tragic consequences of operative failure ending in amputation. Operating on smaller vessels lower down the leg involves a more exacting surgical technique with a higher risk of failure.

Aortoiliac reconstruction

Atheromatous disease of the aortoiliac segment takes three forms. Surgical treatment offers excellent results when atheroma is either limited to the aortic bifurcation, or extends down the common and external iliac arteries leaving the femoral artery relatively free of disease. Successful relief of symptoms is more difficult if the femoropopliteal segment is involved in addition to the aortoiliac region, and may involve both aortoiliac and femoropopliteal reconstructions.

Two main surgical techniques are available. If the atheromatous disease is confined to a localized segment of arterial wall – the aortic or iliac bifurcations, for example – a simple thromboendarterectomy will give excellent immediate and long-term results. Where the disease is more extensive, and in younger patients in whom progression of the atheromatous process can be expected to continue, it is often better to bypass the diseased segment with a synthetic graft.

Endarterectomy

Aortoiliac endarterectomy is a major abdominal operation lasting between 2 and 3 hours. Under general anaesthesia the abdomen is opened through a midline or paramedian incision. After a general examination of the peritoneal cavity to exclude any other serious pathology has been performed, the small bowel is packed away to expose the aorta and its branches. Taking care to preserve the pre-sacral nerves in male patients, the anterior surface of the aorta is cleared above the highest atheromatous plaque. The iliac vessels are also mobilized and controlled. Before any vessel is clamped, total body heparinization is carried out using 10 000–15 000 units of heparin depending on the patient's weight. Once anticoagulated, the aorta and iliac vessels are cross-clamped, and a thromboendarterectomy performed. Having checked that no loose fronds obstruct the lumen of the vessels, fragments of debris are flushed out, and the arteriotomy closed. Removal of the clamps restores arterial perfusion to the lower limbs. If the result appears satisfactory, heparin is reversed with protamine and the abdomen closed without drainage.

Extraperitoneal approach

Occasionally it may be possible to carry out a thromboendarterectomy on a short iliac stenosis using an extraperitoneal approach. Although this takes less time and does not involve a laparotomy, it can be difficult technically, particularly if there are flaps of intima which may dissect on releasing the clamps.

Bifurcation grafts

Aortofemoral bifurcation grafts (the 'piggy back'), while requiring a laparotomy, do not involve so much dissection of the aorta and there is less risk of postoperative disturbances of sexual function in the male. A short segment of the abdominal aorta is cleared and a side clamp applied so that blood continues to flow through the aorta while a Dacron prosthesis is being sutured to an incision in the aortic wall. The limbs of the Dacron bifurcation graft are passed retroperitoneally beneath the inguinal ligament and sutured end-to-side to the common femoral artery on each side. As the patient is usually anticoagulated during these manoevures, the Dacron graft is preclotted with the patient's own blood before heparin is given, so that bleeding from the mesh of the graft is minimal when the clamps are released. Prophylactic antibiotics are given when such a prosthetic graft is inserted to minimize the risk of infection.

Mortality

Aortoiliac reconstruction carries an operative mortality of 2–5%.

Morbidity

About 3% of patients have postoperative complications, the most dangerous being graft infection with secondary haemorrhage or false aneurysm formation, and an aortoduodenal fistula. Male patients may have some disturbance of sexual function unless care is taken during the aortic dissection; on the other hand, some patients find their erectile performance improved with the restoration of blood flow to the internal iliac arteries. The long-term results of aortoiliac reconstructions are good, 80–90% being patent after 5 years.

Femoropopliteal reconstruction

The femoropopliteal segment is the commonest site for clinically important arterial occlusive disease of the lower limb.

Endarterectomy

Attempts to carry out long thromboendarterectomies of the diseased femoral artery, whether by open operation with insertion of a vein patch to prevent narrowing of the artery or by the closed method using ring strippers, were marred by early failure of the reconstruction. While there still remains a place for thromboendarterectomy of a short segment which is occluded or stenosed, the majority of reconstructions involve a bypass graft. The preferred site of proximal anastomosis remains the common femoral artery, but the distal anastomosis has progressed further and further down the leg.

Vein bypass   The patient's own reversed saphenous vein is still the ideal graft. Usually the vein is taken from the same leg and reversed to prevent its valves obstructing the blood flow. Occasionally an *in-situ* vein graft may be used, tributaries being ligated and the valves made incompetent. The groin is explored under general anaesthesia and the common femoral artery together with its main branches is exposed and controlled. The site chosen for the distal anastomosis is then explored to confirm the preoperative radiological findings. Should the saphenous vein be selected it is carefully removed via one or more incisions along the medial side of the thigh and its tributaries are ligated. Local heparin is given before the vessels are clamped and the graft sutured in position. Distally the graft is anastomosed to the proximal vessel which has direct continuity with the foot. Where there is a distal popliteal occlusion, the graft may be taken down to a tibial artery provided it has an internal diameter of at least 2 mm.

Synthetic grafts   The most pressing major problem remains the search for an adequate substitute for the saphenous vein if it has already been removed, or it is found to be too narrow or too short. Arterial homografts and heterografts, together with Dacron prostheses and the Sparks mandrill, are now of historical interest. At present we have available synthetic grafts of expanded Teflon (polytetrafluoroethylene, PTFE) and human umbilical vein grafts.

Results   The results of femoropopliteal reconstructive procedures depend on many factors including the nature of the graft material, the site of the distal anastomosis and the adequacy of the distal run-off. Diabetics do not do so well as non-diabetics, and patients who persist in their cigarette smoking have poorer results than those who stop smoking altogether, but perhaps the most important factors are the clinical judgment and the operative skill of the vascular surgeon.

Patients lucky enough to have a patent popliteal artery with a three-vessel run-off in the calf can expect an immediate post-operative patency rate using autogenous vein of 95%, this excellent result being maintained at 5 years with an 85% patency rate. The further down the limb the distal anastomosis is taken, the more disappointing the results. PTFE and umbilical vein grafts have been reported as having patency rates very similar to those achieved with autogenous vein. Graft occlusion is almost inevitable at some stage, however, either due to progression of the atheromatous disease in the proximal or distal artery, or to some intrinsic defect in the graft itself.

Long-term outcome   When reviewing the results of reconstructive procedures for peripheral vascular disease, it is salutary to remember that from one third to half of all patients undergoing femoropopliteal grafting for intermittent claudication will be dead within 5 years.

3 The critically ischaemic limb

Definition – Clinical features – Management – Results

Definition

Acute critical ischaemia

Critical ischaemia in chronically ischaemic limb

Acute critical ischaemia occurs when the blood supply to a limb is suddenly cut off as a result of trauma, thrombosis, embolus or venous gangrene. In arteriosclerosis, reduction in arterial blood flow following degenerative changes in the vessel wall results in arterial thrombosis with a sudden reduction in any existing claudication distance. The development of rest pain, and impending gangrene, indicate that the limb is in a critically ischaemic state.

Doppler ankle pressures

The term 'critical ischaemia' is used when the ankle blood pressure measured by Doppler is less than 40 mmHg, or the ankle blood pressure is lower than 60 mmHg when there is superficial tissue necrosis of the foot or digital gangrene involving the base of the phalanx. An increasing number of patients with limb-threatening ischaemia are seeking the vascular surgeon's advice. They are often elderly, with other manifestations of cardiopulmonary and cerebrovascular disease, and discussion centres on whether they should be investigated with a view to have a limb salvage procedure or have a straightforward amputation.

Clinical features

Many of these arteriopaths already have evidence of peripheral vascular disease before the onset of the acute episode, and may have been claudicating in one or both legs for some time. A

Decrease in claudication distance

sudden decrease in the claudication distance, or involvement of a more proximal muscle group, often marks the thrombotic vascular occlusion, or the extension of the thrombosis to involve another segment of arterial tree.

Rest pain

Rest pain results from ischaemia of the affected tissues and structures. Pain usually starts in the foot before spreading to the lower leg as the disease progresses. Worse at night, the patient finds initial temporary relief by walking about, but soon resorts to hanging his leg out of bed where the dependent position affords slight relief. Eventually, haggard through lack of sleep, he spends his nights sitting in a chair. Examination reveals a foot which becomes pale on elevation and then turns a reddish-blue colour when placed in a dependent position.

Pressure ulcers

Gangrenous changes occur in the toes and over pressure areas, particularly the heels and lateral aspects of the foot. The initial telltale signs are of a bloodstained discharge from between the toes, or a mottled discoloration of the heel. Before long, one or more toes go black, and the skin of the heel blisters,

Gangrene

breaks down and becomes infected. A zone of demarcation may develop between living and dead tissue if the circulation is adequate, but the appearance of a permanent bluish-black mottling of the skin represents irreversible ischaemia.

Management

It has been said that the competence of a vascular unit can be judged by its amputation rate for critical ischaemia. Whereas in the past, when faced with the situation described above, the general surgeon would have reached for his knife, nowadays, the

Arteriogram

vascular surgeon is more likely to arrange an urgent arteriogram.

When the viability of a leg is at stake, the criteria for advising limb salvage surgery are much broader than for intermittent claudication. Provided the patient can withstand a general anaesthetic (and there are now very few patients deemed too ill for this), and provided that a recent stroke has not made it impossible for the patient to walk again, every effort should be made to save the limb.

Conservative measures are instituted to relieve pain and prevent deterioration of the ischaemic foot while investigations

Stop smoking

are being carried out. Cigarette smoking is forbidden. The patient is rested in bed with the foot in a dependent position,

Cool foot and the limb is exposed and cooled with an electric fan to reduce its metabolic activity. Any septic lesions are cultured and a course of appropriate antibiotics commenced – usually a broad spectrum antibiotic together with metronidazole. Pain is controlled by suitable analgesics. Intravenous naftidrofuryl (Praxilene) has been shown to relieve ischaemic rest pain in controlled trials but it is doubtful if any other so-called vasoactive drugs are helpful.

Antibiotics

Analgesics

Sympath-ectomy At this stage in the progress of peripheral vascular disease, particularly if the arteriogram reveals little scope for reconstructive surgery, thoughts turn to the possibility of increasing blood flow to the ischaemic limb by performing a lumbar sympathectomy. Skeletal muscles are diffusely innervated by sympathetic nerve fibres. The arterioles, however, have a high intrinsic muscular tone which only relaxes in response to an increase in local metabolites produced during exercise. Sympathectomy cannot increase exercise hyperaemia in the dilated muscle capillary bed, although it may have an effect on collateral vessels. An increase in skin blood flow following sympathectomy is also unlikely to be significant as these vessels are also maximally vasodilated by the local metabolites present in ischaemic skin. Lumbar sympathectomy is not without its mortality (about 6%), and has not been shown to confer any benefit to patients with a critically ischaemic limb.

Phenol sympath-ectomy Where sympathectomy may sometimes help, is in relieving ischaemic pain to a certain extent by interrupting afferent pain fibres travelling along the sympathetics. The injection of phenol solution around the lumbar sympathetic ganglia, using a long needle passed through the back under radiological control, may bring symptomatic relief to the elderly patient for whom no reconstructive surgery is possible, and who rejects the advice to have an amputation.

Vascular reconstruction To save a limb, all the techniques and skill of the vascular surgeon come into play. Aortoiliac reconstruction, either by direct surgery or using a balloon dilatation, femoropopliteal or femorotibial grafts, and extra-anatomic grafts such as axillofemoral or femorofemoral crossover grafts may increase the blood supply to an ischaemic limb enough to make the difference between limb salvage and amputation.

Results

The mean survival time following limb salvage surgery is only

2 years, and over 80% of patients are dead within 5 years. However, salvage rates of 70–80% are possible at 1 year follow-up, and even if a reconstruction occludes within a short period of time, the limb very often survives.

When should arteries be dilated?

Percutaneous transluminal angioplasty – Technique – Indications

Percutaneous transluminal angioplasty

In 1964 a technique of passing a balloon catheter along an artery to dilate a blocked or narrowed segment was first described. Ten years later the introduction of a fixed-volume, non-distensible balloon catheter no larger than standard angiographic catheters opened the way for interventional radiologists to take on the management of some arterial problems. Vascular surgeons were far from enthusiastic in encouraging this line of treatment as they knew of the variability in the structure of atheromatous plaques, and feared possible disastrous consequences of any complications. However, the adoption of a team approach in a number of centres with close co-operation between the vascular surgeon and the interventional radiologist now permits a more reflective assessment of the place of percutaneous transluminal angioplasty.

Technique

The technique is relatively simple to describe. Using local anaesthesia, a needle is inserted into the appropriate artery through which a flexible guide wire is passed along the lumen of the vessel through the site to be dilated. After withdrawal of the needle, a balloon catheter is passed over the guide wire and

29

positioned within the lesion under X-ray control using an image-intensifier. The balloon is inflated to 4–6 atmospheres pressure with a dilute radio-opaque contrast medium. After the balloon has been deflated, the catheter is withdrawn and arteriograms taken to confirm that the dilatation has been successful. Direct pressure is applied to the arterial puncture site for a quarter of an hour or so to prevent haematoma formation. The patient rests for several hours and returns home to normal activities the following day.

Effects on atheromatous plaques
Atheromatous deposits vary in their structure and extent, ranging from subintimal plaques containing material the consistency of toothpaste, to ulcers filled with debris or solid calcified lesions. They may be eccentric or circumferential in relation to the arterial wall and extend over a few millimetres to a number of centimetres, causing either a stenosis or a complete arterial occlusion.

With such variation in the structure of the plaque, it will come as no surprise to learn that balloon dilatation causes a variety of changes in the arterial wall. Thus some solid plaques will split, others become impacted into the relatively normal arterial wall, while the contents of softer lesions are squeezed into the layers of the arterial wall above and below the site of dilatation.

Advantages
The advantages of this technique over the alternative of major reconstructive vascular surgery are obvious. A procedure lasting for less than 1 hour, performed using a local anaesthetic with a 48-hour stay in hospital, is attractive to doctor and patient alike, especially when considering poor-risk patients or arterial lesions in anatomical sites difficult to reach by surgery. Tibial, femoral, iliac, aortic, renal, mesenteric, coronary, subclavian, vertebral and carotid lesions have all been dilated.

Vessels dilated

It will be equally obvious that not all lesions are suitable for balloon dilatation, either because of their extent, or because of the risks of complications, particularly of distal embolization to the coronary or cerebral circulations. Of those patients presenting with symptomatic occlusive vascular disease, perhaps one third are suitable for this line of treatment.

Results and complications
The best results are obtained when the procedure is performed by an experienced interventional radiologist using high quality X-ray equipment. In expert hands, the complication rate is less than 5%, but haemorrhage, embolization or thrombosis may occur, and balloon dilatation should only be undertaken by a radiological and vascular service working closely together.

Indications

Iliac and femoral stenoses

In the field of peripheral vascular disease, the most suitable lesions are short stenoses of the iliac and femoral segments. These may be dilated per-operatively to improve inflow to a femoro-distal reconstruction, or as a definitive procedure in high-risk patients. The fact that balloon dilatation does not preclude or compromise the results of any subsequent vascular reconstruction will broaden the indications in this latter group. Successful dilatation does not appear to be a transient phenomenon, and although the follow-up period to date is short, there is now a definite place for this method of treating occlusive vascular disease.

5 Acute ischaemia and arterial embolism

Thrombosis – Embolism – Clinical features – Management

Thrombosis and embolism

Sudden interruption of the arterial blood supply to a limb will result in death of the extremity unless corrected within a few hours. An artery may be occluded by pressure from without caused by a tourniquet or tight plaster cast, from changes in the arterial wall associated with a dissecting aneurysm or trauma, or from an obstruction within the lumen due to arterial thrombosis or embolism.

Aetiology

Thrombosis

Acute arterial thrombosis in peripheral vascular disease may present as an emergency with an acutely ischaemic limb, and very often occurs as a terminal event following acute cardiac failure in the elderly. There is very often a history of claudication to indicate the presence of atheromatous disease, and the gradual development of the clinical features of arterial occlusion contrasts with the sudden onset of symptoms and signs when an embolus lodges in the peripheral arterial tree.

Embolism

Arterial emboli consist most often of blood clots formed in the left atrium of a patient suffering from atrial fibrillation. Another common site of origin is the wall of the left ventricle following a myocardial infarction. Clot may also be dislodged from an aneurysm, and embolization may be the presenting feature that leads to its recognition.

Less common emboli consist of vegetations from heart valves the seat of bacterial endocarditis, or of platelet clumps or atheromatous material dislodged from plaques in the major arteries. An atrial myxoma classically presents as a peripheral embolus. This is exceedingly rare; so is the finding of a foreign body such as a bullet.

Emboli tend to lodge where the artery divides into its branches, the aortic bifurcation, iliac bifurcation, common femoral or popliteal arteries in the lower limb; the brachial artery in the upper; and the carotid or visceral arteries. A saddle embolus can split at the aortic bifurcation with fragments lodging lower down on both sides, while an embolus at one site may fragment and block an artery at its next major branch.

Saddle embolus

Pathophysiology

The effects of an embolus depend on a number of factors, including the level and degree of obstruction and the subsequent development of secondary thrombus, the condition of the arterial wall involved and the degree of development of any collateral circulation.

Tissue death

Once the arterial blood supply is cut off, tissues begin to die, the most metabolically active going first. Muscle, particularly if it has been exercising immediately prior to the arterial occlusion, is the most active tissue and will be irreparably damaged after 4–5 hours' ischaemia. During this period the ischaemic muscle swells, a condition that can easily aggravate the situation when the muscle group is confined within a tight fascial compartment such as the calf. Nerves are also metabolically active and dependent on a good blood supply for their function. Progressive loss of conductive ability manifests itself in increasing anaesthesia and loss of motor power. Skin is the least active tissue and may survive 6–8 hours' total ischaemia. Loss of neuromuscular function is followed by tissue death and, once the skin surface breaks down, bacterial infection of the infarcted tissue results in gangrene. In limbs with a good collateral blood supply, a line of demarcation may develop between living and dead tissue, but when a rampant spreading in-

Muscle

Nerves

Skin

Line of demarcation

Gangrene fection ensues, wet gangrene soon spreads up the limb, often associated with clostridial gas-producing organisms.

Clinical features

The clinical features are not always clearcut, and in about half the cases the diagnosis is uncertain. There may be more than one embolus lodging simultaneously at different levels of the arterial tree and recurrent emboli are not infrequent. The classical Predisposing presentation is found in a patient with some predisposing conditions cardiovascular condition (such as atrial fibrillation or an acute Sudden onset myocardial infarction), who complains of the sudden onset of pain in an extremity which, when and if examined, shows the unmistakable features of an acutely ischaemic limb. Unfortunately, there are too many cases of peripheral embolization, particularly in hospitals and during the night, which are not diagnosed until some hours have elapsed, because nursing and medical staff fail to examine the affected limb in a good light. Diagnosis is more difficult when the onset of pain is gradual Silent with a diffuse distribution, or an embolus is silent, pain developembolus ing later as muscles become ischaemic.

Local signs The details of clinical presentation depend on which vessel Aortic has been blocked. An occlusion of the aortic bifurcation causes bifurcation pain in both legs followed rapidly by numbness, coldness and discoloration from hips or mid-thigh down to the toes, together with loss of power in a similar distribution. Generalized skin Femoral necrosis and gangrene rapidly follow. A femoral embolus results artery in pain in the foot and lower leg, numbness, coldness and discoloration usually limited to the foot. Power may be lost in the toes but seldom completely at the ankle. Axillary and brachial Upper limb emboli cause similar symptoms in the upper limb.

Examination Examination soon after the embolism reveals a pale, cool limb with slight impairment of sensation and power. Peripheral pulses cannot be felt below the occluded artery which may be enlarged and tender. After an hour or so, the clinical picture can be misleading as the patient has less pain, the limb looks a better colour and the temperature gradient is not so obvious. This can lull the unwary into a false sense of optimism. A few hours later still, the true situation is revealed by finding an anaesthetic, paralysed leg, the skin showing the blue-black mottling of irreversible ischaemia.

Not all emboli are associated with the sudden onset of pain, and the differentiation between arterial embolism and thrombosis may not be easy as the clinical features in both conditions are the direct and indirect result of ischaemia. The main pointer in diagnosing an embolus is in identifying its site of origin.

Management

Embolism

Six-hour 'Safe period' — Following a peripheral arterial embolus to the lower limb, the maximum safe time within which the arterial circulation needs to be restored in order to regain full function is about 6 hours. Limbs may be saved following much longer periods of occlusion, particularly if a good collateral blood supply is already in existence and the limb is not rendered completely ischaemic. In the majority of cases, however, any delay in making the diagnosis and arranging definitive treatment ends in disaster with loss of limb and possibly loss of life.

The diagnosis of the site of embolism can be made entirely on clinical grounds. No further special investigations are required, and to arrange an arteriogram merely delays treatment in order to confirm the obvious.

Within 6 hours of onset / Low mol. wt. dextran / Heparin — A patient seen within 6 hours of a major embolus should be relieved of his pain and anxiety. An intravenous infusion of low molecular weight dextran (dextran 40) is started in order to reduce capillary sludging and an intravenous injection of 10 000 units of heparin is given while arrangements are made for operative removal of the embolus. Early anticoagulation is important, as it reduces the risk of propagated clot forming on each side of the embolus and blocking important collateral vessels.

After 6 hours — If more than 6 hours have passed since the embolism occured and the limb is still viable, embolectomy should be undertaken in the young and physically active patient, but conservative measures may be more appropriate in the elderly and decrepit. If the limb is obviously dead – anaesthetic, paralysed with characteristic mottling and blistering of the skin – embolectomy is contraindicated and either amputation or symptomatic treatment advised. One exception to this is perhaps a saddle embolus; here it may be reasonable to attempt an embolectomy, although the chances of successful revascularization of both limbs after 6 hours are unlikely and, in the event, failure usually results in the death of the patient.

Delayed embolectomy — In some patients treated conservatively, the limb remains viable but disabling claudication occurs when they start to walk

36

again. Following confirmation of the site and extent of the occlusion by arteriography, excellent results may be achieved by performing an embolectomy even after several weeks.

Technique of embolectomy   The definitive treatment of an arterial embolus is to perform an embolectomy using Fogarty's balloon catheter. Under a general or a local anaesthetic, depending on the patient's condition, the femoral artery in the groin is exposed, controlled and opened. Through this arteriotomy, the embolectomy catheter is passed up and down the artery, the balloon being inflated in order to draw out any embolic material. Successful extraction of the embolus, together with any propagated clot, is followed by a backflow of blood. The arteriotomy is then closed.

Once the circulation has been restored, attention is directed to the source of the embolus. Patients with atrial fibrillation require long-term anticoagulation because of the risk of further emboli, perhaps to the cerebral or mesenteric vessels. Those found to have an atrial myxoma, bacterial endocarditis, a mural thrombus or aneurysm require appropriate investigation and treatment.

Acute arterial thrombosis

Acute arterial thrombosis, although suspected, may only be confirmed when an attempted embolectomy fails. Very often the

Failed   embolectomy catheter cannot be passed for any distance along the femoral or iliac arteries due to atheromatous narrowing of the vessel wall. In these circumstances there are two alternatives, either to proceed with a major vascular reconstruction the extent and nature of which will depend on the results of an operative arteriogram, or to abandon the procedure and manage the patient conservatively.

Ischaemic limb   Conservative measures include the general management of the ischaemic limb (Chapter 3), the correction of anaemia and improvement in cardiac function, and attempts to lyse the thrombus. Thrombolytic therapy using intravenous or intra-

therapy   arterial streptokinase may be successful and should be followed

Anticoagulants   by anticoagulant therapy.

Amputation in peripheral vascular disease

Indications   –   Technique   –   Results   –   Rehabilitation

Despite all efforts to save a critically ischaemic limb, up to 25% eventually lose a leg, and although this is a major blow to the patient, and sometimes to the surgeon, the performance of an amputation and the subsequent rehabilitation of the amputee should be looked on as a constructive rather than destructive procedure. As the average life expectancy after losing a limb from ischaemia is less than 3 years and, of those that survive, half lose their remaining limb, complications and a prolonged stay in hospital should be avoided.

By reason of the underlying pathology, 90% of patients coming to amputation are over 60 years of age, the greatest number being in their eighth decade. One patient in ten has had a stroke or heart attack, and one third will be suffering from diabetes. Half these patients have had attempts at limb salvage, sometimes with initial success in restoring an adequate circulation to an ischaemic foot with relief of pain and healing of tissues. Other old folk will be physically run-down, both mentally and spiritually demoralized after one or more operations have obviously failed to stop the spread of gangrene.

Indications for amputation

Rest pain
Amputation is indicated if the patient is suffering from intolerable rest pain, there is wet gangrene, and in some cases

39

where reconstructive surgery has failed or has not been possible. The patient with severe continuing rest pain is easily recognized. Haggard through lack of sleep he spends his days and nights sitting in a chair, or if in bed, the ischaemic leg hangs out in the most dependent position. Increasingly potent and more frequently administered analgesics fail to give more than temporary relief. Ischaemic changes in the toes and feet become more obvious as the days go by, the oedema of stasis contributing to the development of wet gangrene. As the skin breaks down, the discharge becomes more profuse and offensive. Eventually fever, tachycardia and mental confusion indicate that general toxaemia has supervened.

Gangrene

Toxaemia

In some patients, the clinical features of frank gangrene are not in evidence although there is constant pain. Investigations including Doppler studies of the ankle pressures and arteriography will have demonstrated that an existing reconstruction has occluded, or that no such reconstruction is possible. These patients may be prepared to take their surgeon's advice that an elective amputation followed by rapid rehabilitation is a more preferable line of management than waiting in increasing pain for some spontaneous improvement. However, selecting these patients needs careful judgement and it is usually wiser to wait until the patient is convinced that his leg is not going to improve and that amputation is inevitable.

Once a decision to amputate has been made, the operation should be performed with the minimum of delay on humanitarian as well as medical grounds.

Contraindication to amputation

It is kinder to manage some elderly patients with progressive gangrene of one or both legs and serious coexisting disease – incurable malignancy or cardiorespiratory problems – symptomatically. After discussion of the problems with their next of kin, adequate analgesics are administered to the patient until bronchopneumonia supervenes.

Amputation technique

The aim of amputation in peripheral vascular disease is to remove gangrenous tissue, relieve pain and obtain primary healing of the amputation scar, and to rehabilitate the patient so that he or she can walk again.

Toe and foot   The lower limb may be amputated at various levels. Filleting a toe involves the excision of all dead and necrotic tissue together with the bone while preserving the surrounding viable tissue which is allowed to fall together without tension. The more formal racquet incision employed to amputate toes which have a normal blood supply is inappropriate in the ischaemic foot and its use likely to be followed by necrosis of the skin flaps, infection of the wound and an extension of the gangrene. Amputation of single toes, although often necessary, sometimes results in deformity of adjacent digits which then become susceptible to pressure necrosis and ischaemic change. Unless there are good peripheral pulses with an ankle systolic pressure

Transmeta-   greater than 40 mmHg, amputation of all toes or a trans-
tarsal   metatarsal amputation is unlikely to heal. Only in the diabetic with ischaemic changes from small vessel disease, or where ischaemic changes follow an episode of microembolization, are such amputations indicated.

Choice of   Amputations at a higher level are below-knee, through-
level   knee, Gritti–Stokes and above-knee. The choice of level has to reconcile two opposing factors. The lower the level of amputation, the easier it is to walk with an artificial leg. A below-knee prosthesis is less cumbersome to wear and full control of knee-joint movement and stability is retained. Against this advantage must be weighed the fact that the more distal the level of amputation, the greater the incidence of failure to heal. Nothing is more demoralizing to a patient than, having faced one amputation, to find that reoperation at a higher level becomes necessary.

Below-knee   Most below-knee amputations nowadays are of the long posterior flap variety. The tibia is divided 14 cm below the tibial tuberosity and a long posterior flap of calf muscle and skin shaped and folded forward to make a loose flap with a reasonably good blood supply. The below-knee prosthesis weight-bears not on the end of the stump, but on the tibial tuberosity and condyles.

Through-knee   Amputations through the knee, although preserving the proprioceptive control by suturing the patellar tendon and hamstrings to the cruciate ligaments, has a high incidence of skin-flap failure as such long flaps have to be fashioned to cover the femoral condyles. Fitting a prosthesis is more difficult as the knee joint has to act at a lower level than the normal leg. The

Gritti–Stokes   Gritti–Stokes amputation overcomes the problem of poor healing of skin flaps by excising the femoral condyles, and attaching

the patella to the divided femoral shaft preserves proprioceptive function, but the problem of fitting a satisfactory knee
joint remains.

Above-knee   An amputation 7–10 cm above the level of the knee joint,
although a more major procedure in terms of operative
mortality, usually heals well. By using a myoplastic technique

Myoplastic   of suturing opposing muscle groups together – adductors to
technique   abductors, and flexors to extensors – proprioceptive control is
maintained. Above-knee prostheses are heavier and more complicated to put on, often requiring the wearing of a shoulder and
waist strap.

Results of amputation

Mortality   Amputation in peripheral vascular disease is not without its
mortality and morbidity. Fifteen per cent of patients will die
without leaving hospital, the mortality of above-knee and Gritti-
Stokes amputation being seven times that of below-knee
amputations. Death usually follows a vascular complication
such as a stroke or heart attack, and venous thromboembolism is
not insignificant.

Morbidity   Infection of the amputation wound by clostridia is a considerable risk in the confused, incontinent patient whose dressing is all too likely to be displaced, with resulting contamination
of the wound. Prophylactic penicillin and skin preparation with
iodine solution reduce the risk of gas gangrene and tetanus. The
incidence of wound infection is reduced by suction drainage of
the wound for the first 48 hours or so.

Delayed   Delayed healing occurs in around 10% of amputees, 8% re-
healing   quiring re-amputation. Attempts to find a simple test to help the
surgeon decide on the optimum level of amputation at which
primary healing can be achieved have not met with much
success so far.

Life   Following an amputation, only one quarter of patients will
expectation   live for 4 years, and every effort is therefore made to rehabilitate
patients as rapidly as possible. The longer the period of time
lapsing between amputation and the ability to walk, the less
likely it is that the patient will use his artificial leg. Some years
ago it was common for more than half the amputees not to walk
effectively with their prosthesis. Since then a more aggressive
multidisciplinary approach has resulted in a greater success
rate.

42

Rehabilitation

Prosthetics

Physiotherapy

Limb fitting

Home assessment

Community support

Outcome

Close co-operation between all members of the rehabilitation team before, during and after the amputation produces the best results. Developments in prosthetics influence the surgeon in the technique and level of amputation he performs, and this depends on regular communication between the hospital and the limb-fitting centre. The active participation of enthusiastic physiotherapists helps to prepare the patient for early mobilization in the postoperative period, including walking in the gymnasium using an inflatable prosthesis. 'Off-the-shelf' pylons are available with minimum delay. Patients encourage each other in their walking exercises at regular classes and a friendly club atmosphere helps towards successful rehabilitation. Before the patient is discharged from hospital, various modifications to his home will almost certainly be necessary, and these can be assessed following a home visit from an occupational therapist and social worker. The patient's family doctor and community services complete the team and support and encourage him at all stages of his illness.

Although 95% of amputees who survive the operation leave hospital, the majority returning to their own homes, one half are subsequently confined to the house because they have no legs or are severely incapacitated as a result of a stroke, heart disease or problems with the remaining limb. However, three quarters of these patients manage to use their artificial leg regularly with the aid of sticks, although their walking activity is confined to the house and garden.

Complications

Phantom limb

Neuroma

Half the patients complain of a phantom limb but become less aware of the absent leg as time passes. The condition is most troublesome in patients who have had an unduly long period of unrelieved rest pain before coming to amputation, and those who have not been warned to expect these symptoms. Occasionally a troublesome neuroma forms in the amputation stump causing local pain and tenderness especially on direct pressure. If conservative measures including ultrasound and nerve blocks with local anaesthetics, phenol or nerve destruction with a cryoprobe are unsuccessful, re-exploration and excision of the nerve at a higher level may be necessary.

7 What is Buerger's disease?

Clinical features – Prognostic factors – Management

'The disease occurs frequently, although not exclusively among Polish and Russian Jews, and it is in the dispensaries and hospitals of New York City that we find a good opportunity for studying it in two phases, namely in the period which precedes and that which follows the onset of gangrene. We usually find it occurring in young adults between the ages of twenty and thirty-five or forty years, and it is because the gangrenous process may begin at an early age that the names pre-senile and juvenile gangrene have been employed.'

Leo Buerger (1908). *Thrombo-angiitis Obliterans: A Study of the Vascular Lesions Leading to Pre-senile Spontaneous Gangrene.*

Although it is nearly 80 years since Buerger first described this disorder, we are little nearer to understanding its true cause, and some vascular surgeons have questioned its actual existence. However, there is no doubt that when all other arteriopathies have been excluded, there remains a group of patients with a clinical disease closely resembling that described by Buerger in 1908.

Clinical features

Male   The patient is invariably a man aged between early twenties and mid-forties who has been smoking more than 20 cigarettes a day

Cigarette
smoker

for many years, and who is continuing to smoke at the time of presentation. Although Buerger noted that his patients were predominantly Jewish, this ethnic prevalence has not been confirmed by later studies, and members of any race may be affected.

Natural
history

The progress of the disease features acute exacerbations and long periods of remission. During an 'attack' the patient complains of severe burning continuous pain in one or more digits, often affecting the toes but sometimes the fingers.

Examination

Examination reveals an intense red discoloration of the pulp and hypersensitivity of the adjacent skin. A blister then appears which sooner or later breaks down to form a punched-out, indolent, painful ulcer which is exquisitely tender to touch. Very often the ulcer becomes infected and local cellulitis is followed by tissue necrosis. Over the next few weeks the surrounding skin of the digit becomes pale and anaesthetic and eventually a line of demarcation appears between viable and dead tissue. As the attack subsides, a variable degree of soft tissue loss becomes apparent which has to be tidied-up surgically, usually by a limited debridement and less commonly by amputation of a digit or limb.

Blister

Ulcer

Necrosis

Remission

Claudication

Raynaud's

Hyperhidrosis

Superficial
thrombophle-
bitis

Between attacks patients often have some persisting symptoms attributable to a peripheral vascular disorder. Many complain of intermittent claudication, about one quarter noting this to affect the calf muscles. Others find they claudicate in the feet and rarely in the hands. Raynaud's syndrome is not uncommon and may be associated with an absent radial or ulnar pulse. Many have excessive sweating of hands and feet. Recurrent attacks of superficial thrombophlebitis, particularly affecting the veins of the upper limb, are significant features. Men with these problems invariably continue to smoke cigarettes.

Investigation

Aortography

Investigation is directed to excluding other arteriopathies, particularly early age onset atherosclerosis. To this end, all these patients have a lumbar aortogram to make sure that there are no proximal atheromatous plaques which could be the cause of their claudication, or which may be the source of platelet emboli causing the ischaemic necrosis of their digits. It was originally thought that Buerger's disease could be diagnosed by typical arteriographic features, but the segmental occlusions of calf

What is Buerger's disease?

vessels associated with tortuous collaterals once thought to be diagnostic can also be found in patients with atherosclerosis.

Prognostic factors

Smoking
Exposed to cold

Many studies have emphasized beyond doubt that patients who continue smoking have the worst prognosis. Similarly, patients who are regularly exposed to cold, wet conditions are more liable to suffer exacerbations. A knowledge of these prognostic factors, together with the natural history of the disorder, enables a rational plan of management to be followed.

Management

Stop smoking

Warm, dry environment

Foot hygiene
Minor injuries

Acute exacerbation

Any young man with the clinical features of Buerger's disease – a history of heavy and continuous smoking from an early age, excessive sweating, migratory thrombophlebitis and episodic exposure to cold – should be advised to stop smoking altogether or be prepared to accept the consequences of almost certain amputation in the future. Where working conditions involve exposure to low temperatures and wet weather, every effort should be made to protect the hands and feet. Seldom is it practicable for a patient to go to a warmer climate to live and work. Attention is also paid to general health, particularly foot hygiene, and any injuries to fingers or toes must be treated promptly.

Once a patient suffers an exacerbation of the disease and presents with an acute attack, admission to hospital is indicated. Smoking is forbidden. General measures include keeping the patient warm while concentrating on local treatment of the ischaemic blister or ulcer. After swabbing of any open wounds for bacteriological culture, the digits are treated by alcohol soaks, which are antiseptic in action, and by evaporation help to cool and dry the tissues. Alcohol-soaked cotton wool pledglets are placed between the toes which are exposed and cooled with an electric fan. Many of these men are suffering from athlete's foot and this is dealt with by the application of appropriate anti-fungal creams.

Surgical toilet

Sympath-ectomy

There should never be any hurry to advise amputation. After a while, as the acute episode subsides and the line of de-marcation becomes apparent, dead tissue is excised or a more formal amputation performed. Traditionally, lumbar sympath-ectomy is advised but, while this helps to reduce sweating of the

47

feet, there is no objective evidence that this operation confers any real benefit.

Summary

Buerger's disease is a disorder of arteries and veins of unkown aetiology affecting young and middle-aged men who are inveterate smokers. Characterized by acute attacks associated with indolent ulceration of digits and eventual tissue loss, the progress of the disease is directly related to the patient's cigarette consumption. Acute attacks are treated conservatively and local excision of dead tissue or more formal amputation advised only when a line of demarcation has developed. Unless the patient can be convinced to stop smoking altogether, further exacerbations with associated tissue loss are inevitable.

Aneurysms

Pathogenesis – Aortic aneurysms – Surgery of leaking aortic aneurysms – Dissecting aortic aneurysms

Types   An aneurysm is a weakness and dilatation of an artery due to a congenital abnormality, an infection of the arterial wall, degeneration within the arterial wall or trauma to the structure of the vessel. Aneurysms may be either saccular or fusiform in shape and affect any vessel in the body. Some sites are more prone to aneurysmal disease than others. The predilection of the spirochaete for the vasa vasorum of the aortic arch and thoracic aorta was responsible for the aneurysmal disease of this part of the arterial tree, happily not seen very often these days. However, there appears to have been a real increase in the incidence

Incidence   of the abdominal aortic aneurysms. Over the past 25 years the Registrar-General has recorded a fourfold rise in the reported deaths from abdominal aortic aneurysms. It seems unlikely that doctors and patients could have missed a central pulsating abdominal tumour, but the diagnosis is not always that easy.

Difficulties in diagnosis   Abdominal aortic aneurysm is 'very often diagnosed when it is not present; and also from the obscure nature of its symptoms, is often overlooked when it is'. Thus wrote Sir William Osler in 1905, and there has been little to change this assessment in the last eight decades. The presenting features of an expanding or leaking aortic aneurysm have been confused with almost every intra-abdominal and retroperitoneal mishap. Two thirds remain undiagnosed on admission and even the diagnosis of a

49

ruptured aneurysm may have to wait for the postmortem examination.

Pathology The elastic and collagen tissue of the aortic wall grow to maturity at adulthood. With increasing age, the intima becomes irregularly thickened and the aortic wall is progressively infiltrated with lengthening, tortuosity and dilatation of the vessel until it becomes aneurysmal. As the pulsatile mass expands, the patient may become aware of pressure symptoms on retroperitoneal and intraperitoneal structures. Laminated thrombus forms in the aneurysmal sac and dislodgment of this clot, either spontaneously or after some muscular effort or abdominal trauma, results in peripheral embolization and the development of acute ischaemia in the leg. Once the arterial wall has weak-

Rupture ened, the aneurysm continues to expand until it ruptures. An expanding aneurysm is often associated with episodes of abdominal or back pain and temporary circulatory collapse from which the patient recovers rapidly. Disruption of the aneurysmal wall into the peritoneal cavity results in immediate exsanguination. Extraperitoneal rupture, on the other hand, produces a large retroperitoneal haematoma, the pressure within which, associated with a period of hypotension, presents a retrievable situation provided it is recognized and promptly treated.

Natural history Abdominal aortic aneurysms rarely follow a benign course, and, untreated, 70% of sufferers are dead within 3 years – compared with 12% of the aneurysm-free population of the same age groups. Untreated, a ruptured aneurysm has a mortality of 100%. The operative mortality of surgery for a leaking aneurysm is around 50%, while that for an elective aneurysm graft is about 5%.

Clinical features The abdominal aorta bifurcates about the level of the umbilicus, and an abdominal aneurysm presents as an expansile, pulsatile swelling in the epigastrium. Sometimes the iliac vessels are also aneurysmal resulting in pulsatile swellings in the lower abdomen. In thin elderly people, an elongated, tortuous aorta lying over to the left side of the midline may appear to be aneurysmal although the lumen is only slightly dilated.

X-rays A plain abdominal film may reveal calcification in the atheromatous aneurysmal wall, particularly clearly seen on a lateral film. This will allow the maximum diameter to be measured and an estimate made of the extent of the aneurysm, particularly important if it appears to involve the aorta above the

50

Ultrasound

Generalised
arterio-
sclerosis

Aneurysms
> 4 cm are
dangerous

origin of the renal arteries. Lumbar aortography does not help in delineating an aneurysm as the aneurysmal sac is usually full of laminated clot through the centre of which lies the channel of blood. The extent and dimensions of the aneurysm can be visualized and measured using abdominal ultrasound or computerized tomography.

An aneurysm is only one manifestation of a diffuse arteriopathy. Over 25% of patients have some features of ischaemic heart disease, while over one third are hypertensive. More than one aneurysm is not uncommon and these are often found in the thoracic aorta, common femoral and popliteal arteries. Coincidental arterial occlusive disease of the carotid, mesenteric and renal vessels and the peripheral arteries is not infrequent.

It used to be thought that an aneurysm of less than 6 cm diameter was unlikely to rupture. This is no longer true, and any aortic aneurysm greater than 4 cm diameter should be considered a potential threat to the patient's life. A careful assessment is made of cardiorespiratory and renal function and evidence of other features of arteriosclerosis is sought before advising surgery. Monitoring of an aneurysm's size is easily carried out using the technique of abdominal ultrasound.

Leaking aortic aneurysms

Diagnosis

Resuscitation

Once an aneurysm has leaked there is often a delay in making the diagnosis, usually attributed to misinterpretation of the clinical observations. On some occasions the doctor fails to note the abdominal mass, while on others the mass may be obscured by abdominal distension or obesity. The main symptom is of the sudden onset of severe constant abdominal pain often, but not always, associated with the signs of shock. Although intraperitoneal rupture leads to almost immediate death, patients can live for some time after a retroperitoneal leak or rupture.

Little time is spent on resuscitating these patients, the aim being to keep the blood pressure low in order to avoid any further increase in the size of the haematoma. The first objective is to relieve the severe pain with pethidine or morphine. Initial assessment at the receiving hospital includes a rapid cardiorespiratory examination, the insertion of at least two large-bore intravenous lines, preferably into a central vein, and the catheterization of the bladder to monitor renal function. Twelve units of whole blood are requested and the patient is taken directly to the anaesthetic room. Here no attempt is made to raise the systolic blood pressure above 100 mmHg. Anaesthesia is induced on the operating table, the abdomen and groins having been prepared and draped and the operating team of surgeon and two assistants being gowned and ready to make the abdominal incision as soon as the patient is intubated.

Surgery

Through a midline incision, the abdomen is entered, the diagnosis being confirmed by finding a small quantity of blood-stained peritoneal exudate and a retroperitoneal haematoma of variable size. The surgeon's first objective is to obtain proximal control of the aortic leak by clamping the aorta above the aneurysm. Fortunately the majority of abdominal aortic aneurysms are associated with an infrarenal aneurysmal dilatation originating 3–4 cm below the origin of the renal arteries. It is possible to apply a vascular clamp at this level, allowing renal perfusion to continue uninterrupted. Occasionally a clamp has to be placed on the aorta above the renal arteries to allow control of the bleeding, but this clamp is removed as soon as possible. Once proximal control has been achieved, the anaesthetist rapidly transfuses the patient with warmed whole blood passed through a filter to reduce the risk of shock lung. Distal control is secured next by clamping the iliac vessels below the aneurysm. When the aneurysm is confined to the abdominal aorta alone, clamps are placed on the common iliac arteries. If, on the other hand, there is an aortoiliac dilatation, or aneurysms of the aorta and iliac vessels, a more distal clamping will be required. Once the aorta and its main branches have been clamped, the aneurysmal sac is incised longitudinally and the atheromatous debris and laminated clot evacuated. Back bleeding from the lumbar arteries and sometimes from the inferior mesenteric artery, if it has not become thrombosed as the aneurysm develops, is controlled by suture/ligation of the origins of these vessels. No attempt is made to remove the aneurysmal sac which is often closely adherent to the inferior vena cava and its tributaries, the iliac veins. A woven Dacron prosthetic graft of suitable diameter is next sutured end-to-end to the infrarenal aorta, using a single continous layer of monfilament synthetic suture material and, if the aneurysm is confined to the aorta alone, the distal anastomosis is made in a similar fashion to the relatively normal diameter aorta just above its bifurcation. Before the distal aortic anastomosis is closed, the proximal clamp is released temporarily to flush out any clot or debris that may have collected above the clamp or be lying within the graft. Release of the distal clamps checks that there is backflow of blood. If there is any suspicion that distal vessels have clotted, balloon embolectomy catheters are passed down each leg to beyond the popliteal artery to clear both femoral vessels.

While the surgeon is carrying out the vascular reconstruction, the anaesthetist restores the patient's circulatory state with whole blood transfusions, supplemented with units of fresh frozen plasma or cryoprecipitate to replace the coagulation factors lost in the retroperitoneal haematoma. Renal function is supported by the administration of a diuretic. Once the graft is sutured in place, blood flow to the lower limbs is restored gradually to avoid a sudden fall in blood pressure associated with re-perfusion of the ischaemic limbs. Lactic acidosis is corrected by the intravenous infusion of sodium bicarbonate solution.

Should the aneurysmal dilatation affect the iliac vessels as well, a longer and more complicated reconstruction is required. A bifurcation graft is inserted, the distal limbs being inserted either into the common or external iliac arteries, or end to side into the common femoral arteries, access to which is obtained by incisions in both groins. The aortic bifurcation or iliac arteries are sutured to prevent bleeding.

Complications
Surgery of this magnitude involves operating times of between 2 and 4 hours. Consequently there is an operative mortality for operating on leaking aortic aneurysms of 50–60%. Most of these patients have manifestations of arteriosclerotic disease affecting the coronary and cerebral arteries – over one third being hypertensive and a quarter having evidence of ischaemic heart disease. Not infrequently there are aneurysms at other sites, commonly in the thoracic aorta, common femoral and popliteal arteries. The complications of surgery are numerous and include problems with renal and respiratory and cardiac function, problems of massive blood transfusion, and ischaemic changes in the colon and the legs.

Contraindications to surgery
Not surprisingly, doctors have questioned whether all patients with leaking abdominal aortic aneurysms should be operated on. Although a policy of operating on all such patients can be defended when the result of not so doing is death, there is no doubt that any prolonged episode of hypotension (systolic blood pressure below 100 mmHg) adversely affects the outcome. Certainly anyone over the age of 70 years, in shock and with concomitant disease, should be allowed to die in peace.

Dissecting aortic aneurysms

Clinical presentation
Dissecting aortic aneurysms are probably more common than we suspect – the clinical features of severe chest and back pain, circulatory collapse and rapid death being attributed to myocardial infarction. The problem is more frequent in patients with cystic medial necrosis, and nearly all patients are hypertensive.

Process of dissection
The dissection commences either in the ascending aorta or in the wall of the descending thoracic aorta near the origin of the left subclavian artery. Once a channel opens in the media, blood spirals around the aortic wall. This dissection can spread proximally around the aortic arch, obstructing the subclavian, carotid and innominate arteries to reach the aortic root. Here

Angina
Aortic regurgitation
Tamponade
coronary arteries are compressed, the aortic valve ring is stretched and made incompetent, or the dissection ruptures into the pericardium causing a tamponade. If the dissection spreads down the thoracic aorta it may obstruct the spinal and visceral

Distal compression
branches by compressing them as they pass through the aortic wall. In this way visceral, renal and iliac occlusion occur. Sometimes the dissection extends both proximally and distally. In its spiral path through the media, the dissection varies in the layer

Rupture and re-entry
it takes, sometimes approaching the adventitia through which it can rupture causing a large haematoma or exsanguination, sometimes bursting through the intima to re-enter the true lumen of the vessel.

Signs
Clinical examination may reveal evidence of hypertension, variable loss of peripheral pulses, raised jugular venous pulse and aortic regurgitation. A left haemothorax, anuria and abdominal pain are of grave prognostic significance. Unless a leg becomes ischaemic following occlusion of the iliac artery,

Conservative management
initial treatment is conservative with bed rest, sedation and antihypertensive therapy to bring the systolic blood pressure down to around 100 mmHg. If the patient survives the acute episode and the dissection has stabilized it may be further investigated by aortography or computerized tomography. Evidence of myocardial ischaemia or aortic regurgitation would indicate the

Surgery
need for urgent surgery to the aortic root, while an iliac artery occlusion requires a laparotomy and a re-entry procedure to allow blood in the false channel to re-enter the true arterial lumen. The results of a more aggressive surgical approach to this vascular catastrophe are encouraging.

What about sex, doctor?

Physiology – Vasculogenic impotence – Prevention of impotence – Surgical treatment of vasculogenic impotence

Successful sexual intercourse requires interest, ability and opportunity. Many male patients, even those of advanced years, with peripheral vascular disease continue to have an interest in the subject together with opportunities for its satisfaction, but the progress of their arteriosclerosis, or the complications of surgical attempts to correct it, may interfere with the ability.

Normal physiology

Neural arcs Three factors interact to produce a normal erection, intact neural arcs, an adequate arterial inflow and competent venous occlusive outflow mechanisms. Stimulation of the glans penis and related areas can bring about an erection and ejaculation in a man whose spinal cord has been transected, thus demonstrating that this response is mediated by a spinal reflex. In the normal man, psychological influences and his emotional state play an important part in initiating sexual activity, and any or many sense organs can be an appropriate afferent stimulus. These stimuli are long-circuited through the higher centres of the brain, where they may be reinforced or inhibited. Efferent parasympathetic fibres via the nervi erigentes relax penile arterioles

55

Venous occlusive sphincters
Arterial flow

and contract the venous occlusive sphincters in the base of the penis. These sphincters do not completely stop venous drainage, as even when the penis is erect some blood must continue to leave the engorged corpora cavernosa. Stimuli resulting from friction of the glans penis, reinforced by other afferent streams and psychological factors, result in a reflex sympathetic discharge via the hypogastric nerves which closes the internal vesical sphincter, stimulates contraction of smooth muscle in the seminal vesicles and prostate, and initiates rhythmic contractions of the ischiocavernosus and bulbospongiosus muscles resulting in ejaculation.

Ejaculation

Types of impotence – vasculogenic impotence

Interference with the sacral parasympathetic outflow or occlusion of the arterial blood supply to the corpora cavernosa prevents erection, while interruption of the lumbar sympathetic outflow via the hypogastric nerves prevents ejaculation.

Poor arterial outflow

Impotence is a well-recognized symptom in peripheral vascular disease when failure to attain or maintain an erection may be due to poor arterial blood flow in the internal iliac arteries. Although young men may be able to have normal sexual function with only one patent internal iliac artery, the older man may notice sexual dysfunction due to diminished blood flow on both sides.

Arterio-sclerosis

As the aortoiliac blood flow becomes diminished, the patient may notice increasing difficulty in achieving or maintaining an erection. Sometimes although an erection is achieved it is lost again during the active pelvic thrust phase. This is

Internal pudendal 'steal'

caused by a steal phenomenon, the other muscular branches of the internal iliac artery 'stealing' blood from the internal pudendal arteries in response to increased gluteal muscle contraction. Other patients notice a sudden and complete loss of erectile

Embolism

function which can be attributed to embolism from the diseased aortoiliac vessels. Diabetics have their own problems – with

Diabetes

both vasculogenic impotence associated with small vessel disease, and a neuropathy interfering with nervous mechanisms.

Assessment

The assessment of vasculogenic impotence depends on obtaining an accurate history from the patient and his partner.

Occasionally special investigations are indicated, including arteriography to demonstrate the internal pudendal arteries.

Prevention of impotence

Surgical procedures are designed to minimize the effects on erectile capacity. The incidence of postoperative impotence has been reported as high as 88%, but there are not many detailed studies on which to base any firm conclusions. As disruption of the hypogastric plexus is known to cause impotence, avoidance of dissection around the origin of the inferior mesenteric artery, preservation of the fibrofatty retroperitoneal tissue over the front of the abdominal aorta, and the left common iliac artery, are now part of the technique in elective aortoiliac surgery. These procedures are often impossible in emergency surgery when the prime aim is to save the patient's life. Care is also taken to avoid embolization of clot and atheromatous debris down the internal iliac system. Interference with the sympathetic outflow in the lumbar ganglia is likewise avoided wherever possible.

Surgical treatment of vasulogenic impotence

Definitive surgery for vasculogenic impotence is seldom performed in this country at the present time, but endarterectomy or balloon dilatation of blocked internal iliac arteries may be useful. On a more ambitious scale, reports of direct revascularization of the corpora cavernosa by a saphenous vein graft from the femoral artery and direct implantation of the inferior epigastric artery have been published.

With a greater understanding by surgeons of their role in causing and preventing problems of erectile function, every man being advised to have elective aortoiliac surgery should have the opportunity of a frank discussion about his sexual activities and expectations.

10 Vascular surgery of the intestinal tract

Anatomy – Pathology – Chronic intestinal ischaemia – Acute intestinal ischaemia

Anatomy

Coeliac axis

Inferior mesenteric artery

Superior mesenteric artery

'Central anastomotic artery'

The stomach, and large intestine are supplied with arterial blood from the visceral branches of the abdominal aorta. The coeliac axis supplies the stomach and duodenum and has numerous interconnecting branches via the hepatic, splenic and left gastric arteries. The inferior mesenteric artery supplying the left side of the colon also has connections with the internal iliac arteries via its middle and inferior rectal branches. The superior mesenteric artery supplies the metabolically active midgut from the duodenojejunal junction to the distal transverse colon, its right colic branch being connected to the left colic branch of the inferior mesenteric artery by the 'central anastomotic artery' which assumes crucial significance in cases of mesenteric ischaemia.

Pathology

Athero-sclerosis

Fibromus-cular hyper-plasia

Thromboangi-itis obliterans

As elsewhere in the arterial tree, the lumen of the visceral arteries may be stenosed or occluded by thrombosis or embolism. Atherosclerosis is the commonest cause of arterial wall degeneration, but fibromuscular hyperplasia, thromboangiitis obliterans and aortic dissection may occlude or compress the vessel lumen. A minor degree of mesenteric artery stenosis is known to occur in the majority of people as they get older, and

59

Aortic
dissection
Embolus

the superior mesenteric artery is partially or completely blocked in two thirds of individuals over the age of 55. Arterial embolus is associated with atrial fibrillation, or the dislodgement of a mural thrombus following a myocardial infarction.

Mesenteric
vein
occlusion

Occlusion of the mesenteric veins is probably much more common than we suspect, and is associated with generalized infections, local venous stasis, intra-abdominal tumours, intestinal volvulus and blood dyscrasias. Mesenteric vein thrombosis has also been reported as a consequence of taking the contraceptive pill.

Natural history

Significance
of arterio-
graphic ab-
normalities

Although the outcome of an extensive visceral infarction is usually fatal, there appears to be no correlation between the degree of mesenteric artery stenosis and previous gastro-intestinal symptoms. Even the radiological demonstration of stenosed or blocked visceral arteries has doubtful clinical significance.

Chronic intestinal ischaemia

True intestinal angina is exceedingly rare, but its ultimate sequel of massive gangrene of the bowel is not. More than half the patients presenting with such an intra-abdominal catastrophe have had suggestive symptoms for hours or weeks before the critical occlusion occurs.

Intestinal
angina

The clinical features of chronic visceral ischaemia are, like those of other arteriosclerotic presentations, commoner in the elderly, the heavy cigarette smoker and those suffering from hypertension and diabetes. Unusually, more women than men are affected. Nearly all patients complain of abdominal pain after meals, weight loss and diarrhoea. Pain is the most common symptom situated in the central abdomen and varying from a dull ache to severe colic. This pain comes on up to 1 hour after eating and lasts between 1 and 4 hours. Unrelieved by alkalis, the patient becomes fearful of eating, loses weight and becomes malnourished. Clinical examination of the abdomen is usually unremarkable.

Arteriography

Arteriography confirms the clinical suspicion, and at least two of the mesenteric vessels are found to be involved. Treatment involves revascularizing two or all three of the visceral

Surgery arteries by the technique of thromboendarterectomy or bypass grafting.

Complications of aortic surgery If there is already existing significant mesenteric artery disease, aortic surgery may well precipitate acute mesenteric ischaemia. This complication follows either aortic grafting for an aneurysm, or insertion of an aortofemoral graft for aortoiliac occlusive disease. Ligation of the inferior mesenteric artery during aortic grafting may have fatal consequences if this artery is the only vessel nourishing the intestinal tract, and recognition of this fact either before or at operation allows the artery to be reimplanted into the aortic graft. Insertion of an Mesenteric 'steal' syndrome aortofemoral graft may 'steal' blood from the visceral circulation, and the possibility of this mesenteric artery steal syndrome should also be recognized preoperatively and dealt with at the time of surgery.

Acute intestinal ischaemia

Acute mesenteric artery occlusion is a catastrophe. The patient, who may or may not have had features previously of intestinal angina, collapses with severe constant abdominal pain.

Pathology The initial pathological changes are those of mucosal oedema which rapidly progresses to necrosis, infection and gangrene. The bowel muscle soon becomes necrotic and ulcerates. Small areas may eventually heal with fibrosis resulting in stricture formation, but massive involvement ends eventually in perforation. An initial intense intestinal spasm progresses to relaxation and dilatation of the bowel as it dies, the gut lumen being steadily filled with fluid and blood amounting to nearly 50% of the circulating blood volume. A bloodstained peritoneal exudate soon becomes a bacterial peritonitis. This 'acute intestinal failure' needs active and urgent diagnosis and correction if the patient is to survive. Apart from a high degree of clinical suspicion, the most useful diagnostic indicator is to find Serum phosphate level a raised serum phospate level. Following urgent resuscitation, a laparotomy is performed. Attempts are made to revascularize Reconstructive surgery the bowel by performing an embolectomy, endarterectomy or bypass procedure as indicated by the findings, together with resection of obviously dead bowel. Should the patient survive 'Second look' operation for 24 hours a 'second look' operation is performed to resect any further segments of dead intestine. The restoration of the circulation to an acutely ischaemic bowel is a major achievement seldom attained in a lifetime of surgery.

61

11 Raynaud's what?

Physiology – Raynaud's syndrome – Raynaud's disease – Raynaud's phenomenon – Assessment and investigation – Treatment

'Madame X, 26 years old, had never been ill; but she had shown since her infancy an infirmity which had made her an object of curiosity among those of her acquaintance. Under the influence of cold, indeed very moderate and moreover the strongest in summer, she saw the fingers become exsanguinated, completely insensible and of yellowish colour. This phenomenon appeared often without reason, lasted a very little time and terminated by a period of reaction which was very painful, during which the circulation became established little by little and returned to the normal state.'

Maurice Raynaud (1862). *De l'asphyxie locale et de la gangrène symétrique des extrémités.*

Maurice Raynaud died in 1881 at the age of 47, the same year in which Sir Thomas Lewis was born. Although Raynaud had postulated a nervous mechanism for the changes he had noted in his patient's hands, Lewis demonstrated the local hypersensitivity of digital arteries to a fall in ambient or body temperature.

Physiology

One of the main functions of the skin blood vessels is to assist in

63

regulating the body temperature. Most of the vessels supplying the body surfaces are under the control of nerves with both vasoconstrictor and vasodilator effects. The digital arteries differ in that they are only supplied by vasoconstrictor sympathetic nerves. In addition to central control of blood flow mediated by the sympathetic part of the autonomic nervous system, digital arteries are also affected by the direct effect of low temperatures. Skin blood flow in normal digits ranges from 0.5 ml/min for each 100 ml of tissue to more than 50 ml/min. Skin oxygen requirements average around 0.9 ml of blood per minute. Thus even in normal individuals it is possible to reduce digital blood flow to a level where tissue anoxia will occur. Intense local cooling of the fingers causes vasoconstriction followed by cold vasodilatation thought to be due to the opening of arteriovenous shunts which allow perfusion to continue.

Vasomotor nerves

Blood flow

Effect of cold

All of us at some time have exposed our feet and hands to low temperatures whether on skiing holidays or while making snowballs with bare hands. The initial pallor of fingers and toes associated with the sensation of cold is followed by numbness due to a combination of reduced tissue perfusion and cold anaesthesia interfering with sensory nerve conduction. Motor function is also affected leading to loss of fine finger movement. On restoration of blood flow, the fingers and toes become reddish-blue in colour, associated with a burning discomfort and swelling of the fingers.

The terms 'vasospasm' and 'vasospastic disorder' are often used in connection with this clinical picture, although normal physiological vasoconstriction in response to nervous or humoral stimuli is not really spasm. However, the terms are now in common use although physiologically incorrect.

Raynaud's syndrome

Some individuals have digital arteries which are much more susceptible to cold stimulus. Raynaud's syndrome is the commonest vasospastic disorder characterized by intermittent attacks of pallor or cyanosis of digits in response to cold and sometimes to emotion. Usually affecting young women, each attack causes the tips of the fingers in both hands to go pale, the pallor spreading proximally to the base of the fingers. The thumb is not usually affected by this colour change. After a variable period of time, the sequence reverses and the fingers go reddish-blue starting at the base and spreading to the tips.

Raynaud's disease

If no other contributory conditions are found to account for these clinical features, a diagnosis of Raynaud's disease is made. The criteria for this diagnosis are as follows:

(1) episodes of pallor or cyanosis of digits on exposure to cold;

(2) bilateral and symmetrical involvement;

(3) absence of clinical evidence of occlusive disease of the main peripheral arteries;

(4) absence of gangrene;

(5) 2 years as a minimum period of duration;

(6) absence of any systemic disease to which the vasomotor changes may be secondary.

Raynaud's phenomenon

Raynaud's syndrome may be associated with, or precede, a number of conditions either affecting the digits locally or the body generally. In these circumstances the patient is considered to be suffering from Raynaud's phenomenon secondary to whichever aetiological process has been diagnosed.

Systemic sclerosis   Raynaud's phenomenon occurs in all the connective tissue disorders but is found most frequently in patients suffering from systemic sclerosis (scleroderma), 90% of whom will suffer from Raynaud's syndrome. It is the arteritis which explains the telangiectasia and Raynaud's syndrome, the vasospasm progressing to digital artery thrombosis and gangrene. The increase in and subsequent degeneration of collagen tissue in the skin and mucous membranes accounts for the thickening and oedema of the dermis and the changes in the gastrointestinal tract, particularly the lower end of the oesophagus. Some patients do not develop progressive systemic sclerosis, but have sclerotic changes in the digits associated with small, painful indolent lesions on the fingers, and are classified as having acrosclerosis. Yet another variety is the 'CRST' syndrome of calcinosis, Raynaud's phenomenon, sclerodactyly and telangiectasia. Thickening of the facial skin and sclerodactyly with pale, long thin tapered fingers with overhanging 'witches' claw' fingernails are the most easily recognized features of this disabling autoimmune disease.

Systemic lupus erythematosus   Systemic lupus erythematosus (SLE) is another collagen disease in which 25% of patients suffer from Raynaud's syndrome. It is the most common and catholic of the collagen disorders, and many systems are involved. Polyarthritis, leukopenia and a positive SLE cell phenomenon are the diagnostic features most commonly found, although patients may present with digital gangrene.

Dermato-
myositis
Polymyositis

A quarter of patients with dermatomyositis and polymyositis have the features of Raynaud's syndrome. The diagnosis is suspected by finding patients with a fever, dermatitis and a myopathy. The light-sensitive erythematous rash is not invariably present. Weak, atrophic tender muscles of the limb girdles and upper arms and legs indicate muscle involvement and the diagnosis is made by muscle biopsy.

Polyarteritis
nodosa

Polyarteritis nodosa affects medium and small vessels of any tissue or organ. Unusual for collagen disorders, it is more common in men and is frequently associated with a peripheral neuropathy and Raynaud's phenomenon.

Rheumatoid
arthritis

In rheumatoid arthritis, as well as Raynaud's phenomenon there is an arteritis which may either (1) take an acute form which is histologically indistinguishable from polyarteritis nodosa or (2) feature a gradual intimal proliferation in the digital arteries.

Sjögren's
syndrome

Raynaud's phenomenon is sometimes found in patients suffering from Sjögren's syndrome in which there is a progressive drying-up of the secretions of the lachrymal and salivary glands.

Buerger's
disease

Thromboangiitis obliterans often involves the arteries of the upper limbs leading to loss of radial and ulnar pulses with severe ischaemic changes.

Digital
artery
thrombosis

Occlusive arterial disease may present some features suggestive of Raynaud's syndrome. Digital thrombosis is not uncommon in middle-aged men. The sudden onset of ischaemic changes in a digit leads to a usually fruitless search for proximal atheromatous disease which may be a source of microemboli.

Cervical rib

Digital artery embolism may be associated with a cervical rib. The long cervical rib lifts the subclavian artery, compressing it against the medial border of scalenus anterior. Haemodynamic changes are demonstrated by feeling the radial pulse, and listening over the subclavian artery while the patient elevates the arms and braces the shoulders back. Loss or reduction in pulsation, and the detection of a bruit, confirm significant interference with arterial blood flow. Any persisting narrowing of the subclavian artery will be followed sooner or later by a post-stenotic dilatation in the turbulent eddies of which thrombus may form.

Vibration injury

Raynaud's phenomenon may be the consequence of a number of traumatic incidents to a digit or the whole hand or foot. For many years, riveters were known to suffer from attacks of coldness and colour change in their fingers, the severity of the attack being related to the amount of vibration the hands were subjected to. Other workers operating hand-held tools have subsequently been identified as being at risk, including regular users of panel hammers, hand grinding tools and chain saws. The vasospastic attacks appear to be related to a frequency of about 125 Hz and are most severe in the digits nearest the source of vibration. Modification to the design of the appliance and the wearing of protective gloves appear to protect the user.

Cold injury

Cold injury to an extremity, whether classified as frostbite, trench foot or immersion foot, can be followed after recovery by Raynaud's phenomenon.

Blood disorders

Disorders of the blood may feature Raynaud's phenomenon. In cold haemagglutination syndrome, red cells clump in those blood vessels exposed to cold. Although the condition is reversible on warming the limb, prolonged exposure to low temperatures results in thrombosis and possible gangrene. Cryoglobulinaemia is another condition found in patients with myeloma and Waldenström's macroglobulinaemia which may present with Raynaud's syndrome.

Assessment and investigation

Any patient presenting with a vasospastic condition of the hands or feet should be carefully assessed, first of all to see whether they really do have the clinical features of Raynaud's syndrome, and secondly to identify those patients who have Raynaud's phenomenon secondary to some other, possibly treatable if not curable, condition. Investigations include a blood count, erythrocyte sedimentation rate, plasma proteins, rheumatoid factor serology, and estimate of presence of cryoglobulins and cold agglutinins. Raynaud's disease is diagnosed only when the criteria outlined above are fulfilled.

Treatment of Raynaud's phenomenon

The treatment of Raynaud's phenomenon is unsatisfactory and no surgical or therapeutic approach has been found to halt the pathological changes taking place in the digital arteries and arterioles, although systemic steroids and sympathectomy may be of temporary value. Chronic ulcers of the fingertip pulp will often heal slowly, and amputation should be avoided.

Treatment of Raynaud's disease

Raynaud's disease seldom requires active treatment. The fact that it has a good prognosis allows the patient to be reassured with confidence that the arterial problem, although a nuisance, is not in itself serious. General advice includes keeping the whole body as well as the extremities warm in cold weather, and working and living in a warm environment. Few patients are in the position of going to live in the tropics! Vasodilators seldom help and sympathectomy has a short-lived effect. An upper dorsal sympathectomy may be indicated in patients with severe and frequent attacks, but although the initial results may be encouraging, within 6 months to a year or so, the attacks return once again.

12 The diabetic foot

Pathophysiology – Clinical presentation – Assessment – Management

The complications of diabetes very often lead ultimately to pathophysiological changes in the feet. These may take the form of disorders of the autonomic nervous system or of the peripheral vascular tree. Add to these abnormalties infection in tissues rich in glucose, and many sequelae appear.

Pathophysiology

The changes found in the arterial tree of diabetics are not specific to the metabolic disorder of diabetes mellitus. These changes are those of atherosclerosis in general, but characteristically occur at a much earlier age and in a more generalized distribution throughout the vascular tree in diabetics. Athero-

Atheroma   matous deposits are found in large and medium-sized arteries, often associated with medial calcification. Small vessels are also affected, the early changes of thickening of the capillary basement membrane being followed by atheromatous deposits in arterioles and postcapillary venules. The development of this

Small vessel disease   small vessel disease, particularly in the toes and feet, accounts for the clinical features of an ischaemic toe in an otherwise warm, well-perfused foot with easily palpable ankle pulses. When diabetic gangrene supervenes, the tissue necrosis occurs distal to the ankle in 90% of cases.

Neuropathy   The neuropathy in diabetes can affect motor, sensory or autonomic nerves. Predominantly it is a sensory neuropathy that is most significant. While the patient is still able to appreciate the sense of touch, that of pain, vibration and proprioception is progressively lost. A motor neuropathy accounts for the wasting and weakness of the smaller muscles of the foot, while loss of autonomic nervous function in the skin of the foot results in loss of skin elasticity and tone.

Clinical presentation

Prevention of complications   Prevention of the complications of diabetes is dependent on good and continuing control of the metabolic abnormality. As in any vascular disease, attention should be directed to trying to reduce the significance of the correctable risk factors. Hypertension is controlled, hyperlipidaemia reduced by diet, drugs or a combination of both, and smoking is condemned. The old, the lonely and the partially-sighted need regular visits and supervision by their medical and nursing attendants, and appropriate help from the community social services. As foot care is so important in preventing complications, readily available chiropody services are essential. All diabetics must be given instructions on the care of their feet along the lines recommended by the British Diabetic Association (10 Queen Anne St, London W1) in the UK, or equivalent national organization elsewhere.

Septic foot   Many elderly diabetics live alone in less than ideal circumstances. Unable to see too well because of their diabetic retinopathy, or to feel pain in their feet because of the peripheral neuropathy, they often present to their family doctor with advanced septic lesions, the presence of which has been recognized by the smell.

Poor healing
Infection   The disturbance in the metabolism is reflected in the skin of diabetics. Wounds are often slow to heal. The appearance of xanthomata and the lesions of necrobiosis lipoidica diabeticorum are related to the altered status of carbohydrate, fat and protein metabolism, while increased susceptibility to infections manifests itself in boils, carbuncles and pyoderma. Once infection has entered the tissues, swelling due to local oedema may impair the arterial blood supply and prevent the development of the vascular phase of the inflammatory response. Staphylococci and β-haemolytic streptococci are common bacterial pathogens, but fungi also play a role in macerating skin, particularly in the toe clefts, and thus break the protecting layer

of intact epithelium. Neurovascular degeneration results in ischaemic and perforating neuropathic ulcers and frank gangrene. The foot is the commonest site of all these skin lesions as it is in the lower limb that there is the highest incidence and severity of arteriosclerosis. Once the peripheral neuropathy has appeared, the patient loses the protective mechanism of pain and trophic stimuli.

Pyoderma gangrenosum
Pyoderma gangrenosum usually follows a streptococcal cellulitis, the skin overlying the most inflamed area becoming devitalized and ischaemic. When the infection has been controlled with appropriate antibiotic therapy, and the diabetic state restabilized, dead slough requires surgical excision, any large residual defect being covered with a partial thickness skin graft.

Neuropathic ulcers
Neuropathic perforating ulcers occur over the weight-bearing parts of the foot or where pressure from an ill-fitting shoe rubs on bony prominences. Most commonly found on the sole of the foot over the metatarsal heads, other frequent sites are over the medial aspect of the head of the first metatarsal and over the head of the fifth metatarsal. Examination reveals an area of thickened, heaped-up hard skin with a central sinus from which escapes a purulent discharge.

Ulcers
Small cracks in the skin and minor traumatic lesions soon become infected and break down into ulcers. Sometimes the lesion is caused by the patient or his attendants. Amateur paring of callosities, overenthusiastic toenail cutting, or the application of astringents, antiseptics or hot solutions, can destroy the protective epithelium. Ill-fitting shoes and walking barefooted subjects the plantar tissues to shearing stresses which may also initiate skin breakdown. All these minor insults, insignificant in normal individuals, are potentially dangerous in the diabetic patient with a peripheral neuropathy.

Neuropathy
The peripheral neuropathy is related to longstanding poor diabetic control. Pain sensation is lost before that of touch and eventually there is a loss of vibration sensation and the ankle reflex. Atrophy of the small muscles of the foot secondary to a motor neuropathy results in changes in the mechanics and stability of the foot resulting in weight redistribution characterised by flatfootedness and hallux valgus. Abnormal shearing forces act on the tissue layers of the sole of the foot, and pressure areas develop redness, hyperkeratosis and eventually super-

Arthropathy
ficial ulceration. Changes of Charcot's arthropathy occur in the midtarsal joints, resulting in clawing of the toes and subluxation

71

of the metatarsophalangeal joints. This deformity may be reduced in the early stages but eventually becomes fixed and rigid. Impaired autonomic function accounts for loss of skin tone with hyperkeratosis and brittle skin.

Vascular
changes
Rest pain
Gangrene

Diffuse vascular changes present with a waxy, shrivelled, hairless foot. Rest pain is rapidly succeeded by the onset of gangrene often following an episode of trauma. The development of moist gangrene is similar to that of pyoderma gangrenosum, with infection and thrombosis combining to bring about tissue death. Dry gangrene on the other hand reflects tissue death with the minimum of oedema and infection.

Assessment

The assessment of a diabetic with a gangrenous toe or foot requires particular care as successful management depends on an accurate judgement of the part played by the three main aetiological factors – infection, ischaemia and neuropathy. A painful,

Ischaemia

cold foot with evidence of pallor on elevation and slow venous filling with dependent rubor is due to arterial obstruction occurring in a diabetic and is investigated and managed primarily as a problem of a critically ischaemic limb. A foot which is

Neuropathy

the seat of a neuropathy is less painful, and infection associated with a degree of ischaemia result in a warm foot with an early spreading infection, the poor blood supply being inadequate to support the inflammatory response.

Infection

Infected gangrene without evidence of ischaemia results in a dangerous situation with pus tracking deep into the foot and, if untreated, up the leg. Due to the neuropathy, the condition is painless, and apart from a general feeling of being unwell, the patient is unaware of the serious nature of his infection which may easily lead to a septicaemia. Assessment of these patients depends on two main pieces of information – the extent of the neuropathy, and the extent of the peripheral vascular disease. Simple clinical techniques of inspection and palpation together with the examination of peripheral nerve function and the presence of palpable ankle pulses will determine the relative importance of each factor. Ankle pressure studies may be misleading, with inappropriately high readings if the calf vessels are calcified.

Management

Ischaemic gangrene is managed as discussed in Chapter 3. In-

72

fected gangrene with neuropathy requires free incision and drainage under antibiotic cover with the expectation that healing will be obtained, although in the neglected case a life-saving amputation may be necessary. In those patients with both a peripheral neuropathy and ischaemia, careful judgement is required to balance the choice between local surgery to remove dead tissue and reconstructive vascular surgery to save a limb.

13 Lumbar canal stenosis

Cauda equina syndrome – Anatomy – Clinical features – Diagnosis – Treatment

In 1911 Déjerine suggested that disorders of the spine could mimic peripheral vascular disease. The spinal cord ends at the second lumbar vertebra, from which level the lumbosacral nerve roots pass down the lumbar canal as the cauda equina, to exit through the appropriate intervertebral foramina. Compression of the cauda equina in the lumbar canal or the nerve roots as they leave it, results in a variety of symptoms which lead the patient to seek advice from a neurological, orthopaedic, physical medicine or vascular specialist.

Definition
The normal lumbar spinal canal has a wide variation in shape and size, and the condition of lumbar canal stenosis is recognized when a variable degree of spondylosis is superimposed on a variable developmental narrowing which combine to produce critical cauda equina compression.

Cauda equina syndrome – clinical features and diagnosis

Leg pain and paraesthesia
The classical cauda equina syndrome is one of pain and paraesthesiae in both legs brought on by exercise and relieved by rest in a patient with normal peripheral pulses. The average age on presentation is between 40 and 50 years, men being more frequently affected than women in the ratio of three to one.

Age

History of back injury
There is a previous history of severe back injury in over 50%. The patient presents with backache, root pain not aggravated by

75

coughing and sneezing, and neurogenic claudication. The symptoms in the lower limbs may be purely sensory with pain and paraesthesiae, or associated with muscular weakness and ataxia. Symptoms are sometimes precipitated by standing with the lumbar spine extended, and are always aggravated by walking and completely relieved by a period of standing still, sitting or lying down. One third of patients complain of some weakness in the legs. Occasionally there is a disturbance of bladder function.

Sensory and motor features

Bladder dysfunction

Examination may reveal transient neurological signs in the lower limbs with weakness of foot dorsiflexion and changes in the reflexes. But the most significant finding is the presence of normal ankle pulses and pressures both at rest and after exercise. Care must be taken in assessing the elderly patient who may have reduced peripheral pulses in addition to a significant but unrecognized stenosis of the lumbar canal.

Neurological signs

Normal ankle pulses

Correct management of this condition depends on an accurate demonstration of the extent and severity of the cauda equina compression. A lateral X-ray of the lumbar spine can reveal a reduction in cross-section of the lumbar canal. Computerized tomography is a valuable non-invasive method of assessing the total cross-sectional area of the bony canal, but radiculography with the injection of water-soluble contrast media is required to demonstrate any compression of neural tissue.

Investigation

X–ray spine

Computerized tomography

Radiculogram

Treatment

The natural history is one of insidious deterioration, eased in some patients for a short time by wearing a corset, particularly if it holds the spine slightly flexed. Definitive treatment requires decompressive laminectomy at the appropriate levels together with other procedures to free any compressed nerve roots.

Natural history

Treatment

The staff of a district general hospital are likely to see 20 – 30 new cases of lumbar canal stenosis each year, of whom 50% will be suitable for decompression. Of these, two thirds are likely to have lasting benefit from surgery.

Results

14 Varicose veins

Anatomy and physiology – Classification – Assessment – Management – Recurrent varicose veins – Superficial thrombophlebitis – Restless leg syndrome

We all know about varicose veins. Many doctors consider them to be rather a trivial if not boring condition, whose treatment is tedious with unsatisfactory results both for the patient and for the doctor.

Anatomy

Long saphenous vein The venous blood from the lower limb drains via superficial and deep veins. The skin and subcutaneous fat are drained by tributaries of the long saphenous vein which runs from the medial side of the ankle up the inner part of the leg and thigh to join the deep femoral vein by piercing the cribriform fascia in the groin. The long saphenous vein is often duplicated, especially below the knee where it has connections with the short saphenous vein and other veins in the leg. Above the knee, an accessory saphenous vein is frequently found in the thigh, communicating with the short saphenous vein and joining the long saphenous vein at a variable level. The long saphenous vein contains 10–20 valves above the knee, but none are to be found lower down.

Short saphenous vein The short saphenous vein passes up the back of the calf, perforates the deep fascia and passes between the two heads of gastrocnemius to join the popliteal vein. It receives tributaries in the calf and communicates with the long saphenous vein or

77

the accessory saphenous vein. The short saphenous vein some-times joins the long saphenous vein in the upper third of the thigh. It contains from seven to 13 valves, one being located at its termination.

Perforating veins

The skin and subcutaneous tissue of the lower leg also drain by perforating veins along the medial and lateral borders of the tibia to join the deep veins of the calf. Valves in these veins direct blood from the superficial to the deep tissues.

Deep veins

The deep veins, which have numerous valves, accompany the arteries and pass between and through the muscles of the calf and thigh. The posterior and anterior tibial veins join to form the popliteal vein which has four valves. The femoral vein contains four or five valves, with one constantly sited just below the en-trance of the profunda femoris vein. There is often another valve just below the inguinal ligament. The profunda femoris vein has two valves below its termination. The external iliac vein is usually valveless.

Physiology

Muscle pump

Within its tight fascial sleeve the calf muscle pump forces blood back towards the heart. At rest in the horizontal position, blood returns to the right side of the heart at a pressure of around 5–10 cm of water. On standing, however, pressure in the deep veins of the lower leg can reach 80 mmHg and, with active use of the calf muscle pump pressures approaching that of the sys-tolic arterial pressure may be reached. Within the deep fascial envelope supported by muscles, these pressure levels are physiological and cause no appreciable symptoms, but loss of efficiency of the deep vein valves, or loss of the protective function of the valves in the perforating veins, result in the transmission of very high venous pressure to the unsupported subcutaneous tissue and to the venous end of the capillary bed. Changes here result in local venous hypertension and sub-sequent alteration in fluid exchanges along the capillary.

Classification

Primary and secondary varicose veins

The term 'primary varicose veins' is used when there is no evidence of venous obstruction. If, on the other hand, there is evidence of obstruction to venous drainage, usually in the iliac or femoral vein, the resulting abnormalities are known as secondary varicose veins.

Varicose veins

Pathogenesis

Valve failure

Over three quarters of patients have primary varicose veins which arise following a local valve failure in a communicating vein between the superficial and deep vessels. The pathogenesis of varicose veins continues to excite argument, but whatever the actual mechanism of perforating vein valve incompetence, once the valve's protective action is lost, high pressure venous blood enters a low pressure venous system. The effect of raised

Oestrogens

oestrogen levels on collagen is thought to be a factor in the development of varicose veins in women who are pregnant or who take oral contraceptives. In other patients, varicosities

Trauma
Family history

appear at the site of trauma, while local thrombophlebitis may destroy a perforating vein valve. Many patients have a family history of varicose veins, and in these individuals there may be an inherited weakness of valve structure, aggravated perhaps by work involving long periods of standing still.

Clinical presentation

Patients may present with (1) asymptomatic, cosmetically unacceptable varicose veins, (2) symptomatic varicosities, (3) the complications of secondary varicose veins, (4) recurrent varicose veins, (5) superficial thrombophlebitis or (6) the restless leg syndrome.

Legs are part of a woman's secondary sexual characteristics and many are upset on discovering that they have varicose veins. Younger women will usually seek advice at an early stage, but housewives and mothers often wait until their children have gone to school before finding time to seek advice and treatment for what they recognize as perhaps a trivial condition. Nevertheless, their varicose veins are important to them when they consider their body image, and the condition deserves to be treated seriously.

Primary
varicose
veins

Primary varicose veins are usually associated with aching legs which tire easily. After a long day of standing, the skin overlying the varicose segment often becomes sensitive to touch, the leg feels unduly heavy and the foot may drag a little. At night the leg becomes restless or cramps develop in the muscles. The foot and ankle often swell, particularly in hot weather or before a menstrual period.

Secondary
varicose veins

Leg ulceration is rarely associated with primary veins, but damage to the deep veins will sooner or later be followed by changes in tissue nutrition accompanied by the development of local oedema, varicose pigmentation, varicose eczema, skin breakdown and infection and eventually venous ulceration.

Bleeding
varicosities
Although venous ulcers do not usually bleed, the skin overlying a large dilated varicosity in the lower leg or foot may become so atrophic that a minor injury is followed by skin breakdown and profuse venous bleeding which, if unchecked, may culminate in the patient's exsanguination.

Clinical assessment

History
Clinical assessment is carried out systematically in a number of stages. The patient is questioned closely about the possibility of deep vein thrombosis and thrombophlebitis. Details of previous surgery or injections for varicose veins are recorded, together with any other symptoms affecting the legs and a note about present and past medical problems. Those presenting with recurrent varicose veins following surgery or injections are questioned about their previous treatment, the indications for it and the initial results.

Examination
The patient is examined with both legs fully exposed, having been asked to stand for a while so that the varicosities are prominent. Secondary varicose veins are excluded by asking the patient to lie down and then elevate the limb. As Trendelenburg pointed out, if the veins do not empty there must be obstruction to venous flow.

Examination of the patient with primary varicose veins is directed to determining which vein is principally involved, and to locating the site of the incompetent valve which allows high pressure blood to leak from the deep to the superficial compartment of the leg. Is it the long saphenous system, the short saphenous system, the lower leg perforators or a combination of them all?

If a normal leg is first elevated to empty the superficial veins and the patient then asked to stand up again, the long saphenous vein fills slowly from below in 25–30 seconds. A varicose long saphenous vein on the other hand fills rapidly from above in 0–20 seconds. The site of the leak may be found by moving a venous tourniquet in stages down the thigh and leg, repeating the filling-rate test in each position. Usually four tourniquet positions are adequate: high thigh, mid-thigh, above knee and below knee. This enables the four possible sites of reflux to be identified. The commonest site of valve incompetence is at the saphenofemoral junction in the groin. Lower down the leg, the other sites are a mid-thigh perforator, an above-knee perforator and a below-knee perforator.

Varicosities of the short saphenous system are less common. They are made more prominent by an above-knee tourniquet and controlled by one placed below the knee. The leak always arises at the site of an incompetent valve at the saphenopopliteal junction. There are no other significant perforators connecting with the short saphenous vein.

In some patients, varicosities appear to be confined to the lower leg and can be controlled by local pressure at the site of the incompetent perforator.

Management

Aims The aim in treating varicose veins is to eradicate detectable varicosities, deal with incompetent perforators and minimize the chance of recurrence while avoiding unsightly scars and other complications.

Elastic stockings A pair of well-fitting elastic stockings may well relieve symptoms in those patients who are not anxious to consider a more permanent cure, or who through age or infirmity are not considered suitable for either surgery or compression sclerotherapy.

Mini-injections Small dilated veins or venules, the 'spiders' which appear on the lower leg and thighs of many women as they grow older, may be sclerosed. As each venule has to be treated separately, the technique demands a good eye, a steady hand, and considerable patience on the part of the injector. Occasionally a well-placed injection leads to a gratifying large area of blanching as the sclerosant reaches a number of interconnecting venules, but extravasation results in an area of tissue necrosis and subsequent ulceration.

Modifications to the usual technique of compression sclerotherapy are required. The usual sclerosant, sodium tetradecyl sulphate (STD) 3%, is diluted with sterile water to make a 1% solution which is less likely to cause ulceration if injected outside the vein. With such small venules to deal with, a size 30 SWG needle is used and magnifying spectacles are a useful aid for the hypermetropic doctor. The 1% STD solution is drawn up into a 1 ml syringe so that small volumes under low pressure can be injected into the dilated venules, 0.1–0.2 ml often being sufficient, although more may be injected if a large area of skin blanches. A cotton wool ball is placed over the injection site and held in place with non-allergic tape. Usually 7 days of compression are adequate, and although leg bandaging is unnecessary, a full-length elastic stocking helps to keep the dressings in place.

Compression sclerotherapy   Varicose veins of the lower leg due to below-knee incompetent perforating veins, or residual veins following surgery, are treated by a course of compression sclerotherapy (Chapter 15).

Surgery   Surgery is indicated when there is evidence of saphenofemoral or saphenopopliteal incompetence. Incompetent thigh perforators in women with fat thighs and large clusters of unsightly varicose veins are best dealt with surgically.

Trendelenburg's operation   Saphenofemoral incompetence is corrected by Trendelenburg's operation. Exposure of the saphenofemoral junction through an incision in the groin allows all the tributaries of the long saphenous vein together with any veins draining directly into the femoral vein to be ligated and divided.

Long saphenous stripping   Incompetent thigh perforators are usually ablated by stripping the long saphenous vein from the medial side of the knee to the groin. It is unnecessary to strip the long saphenous vein from the ankle as the lower part of the vein is not directly connected to the perforating veins of the calf, and the passage of the stripper head is likely to avulse the lower part of the saphenous nerve, resulting in anaesthesia and paraesthesia of the skin over the medial side of the ankle and foot.

Saphenopopliteal ligation   Saphenopopliteal ligation sometimes requires an extensive dissection in the popliteal fossa because of the anatomical variations in the termination of the short saphenous vein, but it is unnecessary to strip the short saphenous vein.

Cockett's operation   Cockett's operation to ligate incompetent perforators in the calf is usually reserved for those patients whose venous ulcers have not responded to compression sclerotherapy. Since the procedure involves a long incision on the medial side of the leg through oedematous and fibrosed tissue, the wound is susceptible to infection, breakdown and delayed healing, even when the gentlest technique is used and the perforating veins ligated below the deep fascia. The incision is often extended to include excision of the associated venous ulcer which is subsequently grafted.

Ligation, avulsion and excision   Large clusters of varicose veins not suitable for stripping may be excised or avulsed. Excision involves fairly long incisions with tunnelling and dissection of the varicosities. Avulsion techniques vary, but by making a number of very small incisions in Langer's line, segments of vein can be mobilized and avulsed with forceps, leaving an insignificant scar.

Postoperative care   At the completion of the operation, the leg is bandaged to minimize haematoma formation, especially when veins have been avulsed. The patient is encouraged to walk on the first post-operative day, returns home on the third day and discards any bandages after a week. Normal household activities are carried out at this time, and unrestricted work and play after 3 weeks.

Recurrent varicose veins

Inadequate assessment

Imperfect surgical technique

Abnormal anatomical arrangements   There are three main causes of recurrent primary varicose veins: (1) the preoperative assessment may have been inadequate or the conclusions drawn from the findings were incorrect, (2) an imperfect surgical technique failed to achieve the objectives, particularly in carrying out a saphenofemoral or sapheno-popliteal ligation or (3) an abnormal anatomical arrangement may have left the patient with two long saphenous veins in the leg, only one of which was stripped out.

Venography   Apart from those with minor trivial varicosities which can be tidied-up by injections, patients with recurrent varicose veins should be investigated by venography either before or during surgery. In this way the actual venous connections can be identified.

Corrective surgery   Surgical treatment involves performing the correct operation, or completing the inadequate one.

Superficial thrombophlebitis

Aetiology   Superficial thrombophlebitis is not uncommon in patients with varicose veins. Most episodes follow minor trauma to a segment of vein which becomes inflamed, the patient noticing the development of a red tender swelling along the course of a vein, followed later by an area of surrounding cellulitis. Occasionally, superficial thrombophlebitis is infective in origin, associated with an infected patch of eczema or venous ulcer.

Treatment   Treatment of superficial thrombophlebitis tends to be rather empirical – the patient is told either to rest or exercise, the leg is either bandaged or left unsupported, and antibiotics or anti-inflammatory drugs may or may not be prescribed.

A more rational approach is to consider the risk of complications particularly of thrombosis spreading from the superficial veins to the deep veins, either via the perforating veins in the calf or at the saphenofemoral junction.

The first question that needs answering is – is there any

evidence of existing varicose veins? If the answer is no, Doppler ultrasound examination of the long saphenous vein will reveal whether this vessel is blocked or not. If the long saphenous vein is patent, the problem is one of a local cellulitis which will respond to antibiotic therapy. If, on the other hand, the long saphenous vein is occluded, the next question is – is the inflammatory process nearing the saphenofemoral junction in the groin? If the answer is no, the phlebitis can be managed with anti-inflammatory drugs. If the phlebitis is close to the groin, study of the deep veins with the Doppler ultrasound will indicate whether they are normal or not. If the deep veins are normal, the saphenofemoral junction needs ligating; if there is evidence of an existing deep vein thrombosis, the patient should be anticoagulated.

The management of patients with existing varicose veins depends on whether the phlebitis is near the groin – if not, prescribe anti-inflammatory drugs. If it is near the groin – ligate the saphenofemoral junction if the deep veins are patent, or anticoagulate the patient if there is evidence of deep vein thrombosis.

Summary   In summary, there are four main lines of treatment of superficial thrombophlebitis:

(1) antibiotics if the main problem is a cellulitis rather than a thrombosis,

(2) anti-inflammatory drugs if phlebitis is confined to an unimportant small segment of superficial vein,

(3) surgical interruption of the long saphenous vein if the thrombophlebitis is near the saphenofemoral junction,

(4) anticoagulation if both superficial and deep veins are involved.

Restless leg syndrome

Symptoms   Over 300 years ago an English neurologist, Thomas Willis, described a condition with the following features – an 'aching, crawling, restless discomfort that starts when the legs are at rest, usually at night, and relieved when the legs are moved'. This syndrome is not uncommon and occurs in all age groups, the majority being between 40 and 60 years. The clinical features are much as Willis described them. There is an aching numbness, or burning tightness in the legs with a heavy tired feeling which is only noted when the legs are still. Very often both legs become restless, associated with spontaneous jerking, jumping or twitching of the same muscle group in both legs. Although the symptoms are most noticeable when the patient goes to bed at night and may prevent sleep, they sometimes become noticeable while sitting in a chair. The symptoms are almost immediately relieved by movement, the patient getting up and walking about, or stretching and rubbing the affected parts of the leg.

Aetiology   The aetiology of the restless leg syndrome is unknown. Often associated with a long period of standing, the syndrome is frequently found in patients with other features of tension, stress and depression.

Treatment   In those whose symptoms are brought about by prolonged standing, almost complete prevention can be guaranteed by wearing a pair of elastic stockings during the day. Drug therapy is usually confined to the offering of analgesics and occasionally tranquillizers. Although deep venous hypertension has been postulated as an aetiological factor in this syndrome, specific drugs have not been shown to relieve the symptoms significantly.

Conclusion

In order to achieve consistently good results in the treatment of varicose veins, a complete and accurate assessment of the venous abnormality needs to be followed by appropriate surgery, compression sclerotherapy (Chapter 15) or a combination of both.

15 Compression sclerotherapy for varicose veins

Patient selection – Injection technique – Complications

The best method of treating varicose veins has not yet been defined. Whenever experts advocate different approaches to the same subject, it almost certainly means that one technique is no better than another. In the treatment of varicose veins, compression sclerotherapy, surgery or a combination of both have a part in relieving symptoms and improving the cosmetic appearance of the leg.

Historical note — Doctors have been injecting varicose veins for over 100 years, but until relatively recently the results were disappointing, with the production of a painful, tender area of localized thrombophlebitis at the injection site, the risk of involvement of the deeper veins of the leg in the thrombotic process, and the recanalization of the thrombus after a few months – leaving the patient's leg in much the same condition as before treatment, if not worse.

Modern approach — Twenty years ago Fegan put the technique of 'compression sclerotherapy' onto a more scientific basis when he pointed out that merely injecting a sclerosant into an uncompressed vein causes a local thrombosis. Although capillaries and fibroblasts advance into the thrombus as part of the inflammatory response in the vein wall, once in an upright position, the 'water hammer' effect of the column of blood in the patient's varicose vein would soon separate the clot from the vein wall and recanalization ensue. However, if the sclerosant is allowed to act for 30–60 seconds on an isolated segment of empty vein which is then compressed for 6 weeks, a fibrous union, or 'endo-sclerosis', takes place with complete obliteration of that segment of vein. Sclerosis of an incompetent perforating vein will seal any leaks through the deep fascia, restoring the efficiency of the muscle pump and often allowing secondarily dilated superficial varicose veins to shrink to a normal size and tone.

Patient selection

Advantages and disadvantages
The advantages of compression sclerotherapy are the avoidance of a surgical procedure with resulting wound discomfort, visible scars and a variable time off work, compared with an out-patient procedure and the convenience of continuing with normal work and social activities. Compression sclerotherapy is not entirely without drawbacks, however. Many patients find a period of leg bandaging for 6 weeks particularly uncomfortable and irksome, particularly in warmer weather.

Contraindications
The clinical assessment of patients with varicose veins has already been detailed above (Chapter 14). Injections in the region of the saphenofemoral junction are contraindicated and in the popliteal fossa unwise; above the knee it is difficult to maintain the necessary compressing bandage in position for 6 weeks. Patients with the post-thrombotic syndrome, or a previous history of deep vein thrombosis, need careful assessment before being advised to have a course of compression sclerotherapy (see Chapter 17).

Obesity
Many women seeking treatment for their varicose veins are overweight. It is important to emphasize to them the necessity of losing weight, and to withhold treatment until they have reduced their weight to within 10% of the average for age and height. The best results are obtained in primary varicose veins occurring below the knee associated with incompetent perforators in the lower leg. Modern formula-

Contraceptive pill
tions of oral contraceptives are not sufficiently thrombogenic to justify stopping the pill in order to complete a course of compression sclerotherapy. The complications of pregnancy are greater than those of injection treatment for varicose veins.

Technique

Identification of 'blow-outs'
The patient is first examined standing and, by using a combination of palpation and percussion, the main varicosities are identified and marked accurately on the leg with a skin pencil or felt-tip pen. The patient then lies flat on a couch and the leg is palpated. It is often possible to feel pits and depressions in the

subcutaneous tissue and these are marked accurately on the skin with circles. Whether these pits represent the actual sites of incompetent perforators coming through the deep fascia, or mere lacunae in the fat of the subcutaneous tissue, is probably academic. In practice, the injection of a sclerosant at these sites will achieve the same result. Either the incompetent perforator will be sealed, or the prominent vein troubling the patient will be occluded. Very often a single perforator is suspected as being the main cause of the varicose vein. By occluding this vein with a thumb and asking the patient to stand again, the suspicion can be confirmed if there is no immediate filling of the varicosity until the occluding thumb is removed. Ultrasonographic localization of incompetent perforators adds a more scientific dimension to this stage of assessment.

Injection technique
With the patient lying flat on a couch, take a 2 ml syringe fitted with 16 mm 25 SWG needle containing sodium tetradecyl sulphate (STD) 3% in the right hand. Enter the skin at a previously marked site and aspirate venous blood to confirm that the needle is in a vein. Place the middle finger and thumb of the left hand 5 cm apart to span and compress the vein above and below the injection site. Inject 0.25–0.5 ml of STD 3% into the vein and, leaving the needle *in situ*, maintain this position for 30–60 seconds depending on the size of the vein to be sclerosed. During this interval there are opportunities to exchange pleasantries with the patient and nursing staff, to explain the procedure and its follow-up, or in well-equipped varicose vein clinics to listen to appropriate background music.

Compression
The next stage is to compress the vein so that blood is expressed from the injected segment and the sclerosed endothelial surfaces are approximated. The aim is to achieve fibrosis of the vein rather than thrombosis of its contents. Various methods of compression are in use, including small sorborubber or plastic foam pads and dental rolls, but the ubiquitous cotton wool ball held in place by a 5 inch (125 mm) piece of non-allergic tape and an assistant's finger is satisfactory. The previously marked veins are injected one by one, a second assistant coming to help as more and more fingers are used up compressing the cotton wool balls.

Bandaging
After one leg has been injected it is bandaged from toes to above the highest injection site. In the majority of patients this will be just below the knee. A 4 inch (10 cm) crepe bandage is applied with a 4 inch (10cm) elastocrepe bandage on top of this. Care is taken not to have too many turns around the ankle and to

avoid any ridges or rucking-up of the bandage. The patient will have to wear the bandages for 6 weeks and during this time compression of the sclerosed veins needs to be constant in order to achieve a sound fibrous union. A spiral of ¼ inch (6 mm) zinc oxide plaster over the elastocrepe bandage will stop the bandage from slipping. A below-knee tubular bandage is placed over

Post-injection walking

these bandages. Before leaving the clinic, the patient is advised to have a brisk walk in order to minimize the effect of any sclerosant which may have entered the deep veins, to avoid standing still and to walk at least 3 miles (5 km) a day.

One-week check

The patient is seen again 1 week later. All the bandages and cotton wool balls are removed and the injection sites inspected and palpated. Successful injection sites feature a small non-tender nodule. At this '1-week' visit, sites of unsuccessful injections at the first visit are reinjected together with any other veins that have not been sclerosed. During these procedures the patient is kept lying flat on a couch until the cotton wool balls have been replaced on all injection sites, and the three layers of bandages reapplied.

Five-week check

Five weeks later the patient attends for a final assessment, having been told to remove all bandages and to take a much needed bath before coming to the clinic.

Complications

Failure to compress a below-knee perforator effectively sometimes results in a chemical phlebitis running up the long saphenous vein in the thigh. The application of an above-knee tubigrip bandage for the first week will prevent this from happening. Patients are often anxious about the residual nodule

Residual nodule

at the injection sites, but may be reassured that these nodules are the result of a successful injection and will slowly absorb over a period of time. Occasionally a segment of vein between two injection sites becomes thrombosed. By the time this is noted, the

Thrombosed veins

thrombosed blood has liquefied and the fluctuant segment can be aspirated with a syringe fitted with a large bore needle.

Superficial ulceration

Although not particularly painful in themselves, injections of sclerosant can cause tissue irritation and even superficial ulceration if the sclerosant extravasates or is injected outside the

Thrombo-phlebitis

vein. Local thrombophlebitis is associated with tender nodularity along the course of the vein, and sometimes pigmentation

Pigmentation

of the overlying skin which may persist for many months. Rarely,

Hairgrowth

increased hairgrowth appears around the injection site. This is

90

Deep vein
thrombosis

Intra-arterial
injection

confined to the area of skin most damaged by the venous incompetence, and could be due to an improvement in tissue nutrition. Although some sclerosant does enter the deep venous system, deep vein thrombosis as a complication of compression sclerotherapy is rare provided the patient walks vigorously immediately after the legs have been bandaged, and continues to walk about 3 miles a day. One particularly tragic consequence follows inadvertent intra-arterial injection of sclerosant into the posterior tibial artery while attempting to inject a perforating vein behind the medial malleolus. The sclerosant has little effect on larger vessels and does not appear to cause any arterial intimal damage or spasm but, in the smaller arteries it denatures the blood into a sludge which obstructs the microcirculation leading to proximal stagnation, secondary thrombosis and eventual tissue necrosis. The patient complains of pain in the forefoot which turns pale and then becomes cyanosed. Immediate injection of intra-arterial heparin (5000 units) and papaverine, followed by systemic anticoagulation and the use of vasodilators may retrieve the situation, but gangrene frequently requires amputation of the toes, forefoot or even the lower leg.

Conclusion

Injecting varicose veins can be time-consuming, and consistent good results can only be achieved by attention to detail during all stages of treatment.

16 Venous thromboembolism

*Pathogenesis – Prevention of deep vein thrombosis (DVT) –
Clinical features of DVT – Management of DVT – Recurrent DVT
– Pulmonary embolism*

Pathogenesis

Historical note   While John Hunter recognized that inflammation in the walls of
veins preceded changes within the lumen, it was the great
German pathologist Virchow who enunciated the now well-
recognized fact that venous thrombosis may be initiated by
changes in the structure of the blood, changes in the wall of the
vein and reduction in blood flow. Later studies revealed that the
process of thrombosis is initiated by a collection of platelets to
which becomes attached and enmeshed a coralline thrombus.
Once the vessel is occluded a propagated clot extends along the
vessel in both directions. Particularly dangerous is the tail of clot
occurring in a larger vein. This tail can build up in only a few
hours, and if broken off is swept along the venous circulation
through the right side of the heart to lodge as an embolus in the
branches of the pulmonary artery.

Early   For many years early mobilization of the postoperative
mobilization   patient has been recognized as being an important factor in reducing the incidence of deep vein thrombosis in surgical wards.
A similar practice is equally successful in preventing deep vein
thrombosis in women after childbirth. Medical patients, however, are often more difficult or impossible to mobilize

adequately due to their cardiorespiratory or other chronic diseases.

Lines of investigation
Over the years a number of attempts have been made to modify the factors predisposing to venous thrombosis described by Virchow. All three factors have been investigated and there have been attempts to reduce clotting by reducing the coagulability of the blood, attempts to reduce platelet stickiness to prevent the initiation of the thrombotic process, and efforts to minimize damage to the vein wall and to maintain a rapid venous return from the legs.

[125]I fibrinogen uptake
Investigation of the different approaches to preventing deep vein thrombosis is mostly dependent on the ^{125}I fibrinogen uptake test. After loading the thyroid gland with an oral dose of potassium iodide, fibrinogen labelled with radioactive iodine is injected into the circulation, and its concentration in the lower limbs measured at regular intervals with a scintillation counter. Should thrombosis take place, a higher radioactive count will be detected over the affected site. This technique can only be applied as a screening investigation, or to monitor the effect of various lines of approach in reducing the incidence of deep vein thrombosis, as the ^{125}I-labelled fibrinogen has to be given before any thrombus has formed.

Prevention of deep vein thrombosis (DVT)

A number of trials have confirmed that low dose heparin, intermittent external compression of the calf, oral anticoagulant therapy commencing preoperatively or at the time of operation, or low molecular weight dextran are effective in preventing deep vein thrombosis. The evidence that these techniques reduce the incidence of pulmonary embolism, although suggestive, is not so convincing statistically.

Low dose heparin
Low dose heparin, 5000 units in a volume of 0.2 ml is injected into the subcutaneous tissue of the abdominal wall 2 hours before surgery, and repeated every 8 or 12 hours until the patient is fully ambulant. In practice this means when the patient is discharged home. With the 12-hourly regimen there has been no evidence of excessive bleeding. The 8-hourly regimen has been shown to be more effective in high risk patients, particularly those with malignant disease, but there is a slight increase in the risk of haematoma formation. Low dose heparin reduces the incidence of ^{125}I-fibrinogen-detectable calf

vein thrombi, reduces the incidence of proximal vein thrombi and also reduces the incidence of major pulmonary emboli.

Calf muscle stimulation

By intermittently squeezing the calves, the technique of external pneumatic compression stimulates the calf muscle in the recumbent patient, thus preventing venous stasis in the sinusoids of the calf. The device consists of an inflatable splint placed over the leg which is intermittently inflated and deflated pneumatically. The techique may be used preoperatively, while the patient is undergoing surgery (provided it is not leg surgery), and continued on return to the ward. High risk patients may be further protected by commencing anticoagulants when safe to do so. External pneumatic compression has been proved to reduce the incidence of deep vein thrombosis, but its efficacy in reducing the incidence of pulmonary embolism is not yet confirmed.

Oral anticoagulants

Oral anticoagulants are effective when the prothrombin time is doubled, but this is often an unacceptable level at which to undertake major surgery because of the risk of operative and postoperative haemorrhage. Doubling the prothrombin time preoperatively has been proved to prevent the occurrence and extension of deep vein thrombi, but this is not so effective if anticoagulation is delayed to the postoperative period.

I.V. dextran

Intravenous dextran, both dextran-70 and dextran-40, is effective in reducing the incidence of deep vein thrombosis. An intravenous infusion of 500 ml dextran is given over 4–6 hours and repeated daily for between 2 and 5 days. There is a slight risk of increased operative bleeding, but the hazard is of overloading the circulation in the elderly.

Choice of agent

The choice of a prophylactic agent against deep vein thrombosis depends on its efficacy, its freedom from significant complication or side-effects and its feasibility. It is also useful to consider which procedures or groups of patients are at particular risk from thrombosis. If we look at patients about to undergo abdominal surgery, a low risk category would include those under 40 years of age, with no history of a previous deep vein thrombosis, having an operative procedure lasting less than 30 minutes, following recovery from which they would be ambulant at an early stage. A high risk patient, on the other hand, would be one with a recent history of thromboembolism, a diagnosis of malignancy, undergoing extensive pelvic or abdominal surgery.

Risk factors in surgery

In the low risk patient, the chance of calf vein thrombosis occurring is less than 3%, of a proximal vein thrombosis or pulmonary embolism less than 1% and of a fatal pulmonary embolism less than 0.01%. In a high risk patient, on the other hand, the incidence of calf vein thrombosis is 30–60%, of proximal vein thrombosis or pulmonary embolism 6–12% and of a fatal pulmonary embolism 1–2%.

Clinical features of DVT

Clinical diagnosis unreliable

The clinical diagnosis of a deep vein thrombosis is unreliable, and the bedside assessment of the presence or absence of a DVT will be wrong in 50% of cases. The classical presentation of a 10th-day postoperative patient with a low-grade fever, pain and swelling in the calf, and a positive Homans' sign on passive dorsiflexion of the ankle is infrequent. Although the value of careful clinical examination and assessment cannot be dismissed, the clinician must have a high index of suspicion and be prepared to investigate further any patient with localized swelling and tenderness of the soleus muscle, apart from the more florid examples of calf or ileofemoral vein thrombosis.

Investigation

Doppler ultrasound

The confirmation of deep vein thrombosis depends on one non-invasive and one invasive technique. Using the Doppler ultrasound, an experienced observer can correctly diagnose a significant deep vein thrombosis in nearly every case. Ascending venography allows a definitive diagnosis to be made, the location and extent of the thrombus to be localized and the existence of a significant extension into the main venous channel revealed.

Management of DVT

Heparin

Once a clinical diagnosis of deep vein thrombosis is made, it is usually wise to start an intravenous infusion of heparin while organizing further investigations to confirm the diagnosis. Non-invasive screening using Doppler ultrasound will produce a normal, equivocal or abnormal result. If there is no evidence of obstruction to popliteal venous flow, no further anticoagulant treatment is indicated and the painful calf can be treated symptomatically with strapping and an anti-inflammatory analgesic, and the patient encouraged to walk. Should the Doppler ultra-

Venography

sound examination be equivocal, venography will confirm or refute the diagnosis. With an abnormal Doppler assessment, a preceding episode of calf trauma warrants venography before committing the patient to a full anticoagulant regimen. With no such history, the Doppler findings of reduction of popliteal venous flow may be taken as accurate and anticoagulation therapy continued.

Admission to hospital
Any patient in whom a diagnosis of deep vein thrombosis has been made should be admitted to hospital where anticoagulant therapy and its monitoring are most easily supervised. Deep vein thrombosis brings about an activation of the coagulation cascade with the generation of large concentrations of thrombin. Low dose heparin is inadequate to control this clotting process, and a loading dose of 200 u/kg body weight of heparin is infused intravenously followed by a maintenance dose of intravenous heparin adjusted to keep the activated partial thromboplastin time between 80 and 90 s (2–2½ times the control value). The fact that heparin has a half-life of 60–90 min justifies the use of a continous intravenous infusion rather than bolus intravenous injections. Depending on the extent and site of the thrombus, intravenous heparin is continued for 10–14 days, following which the patient may either be returned to a low dose heparin regimen or started on an oral anticoagulant.

Warfarin
A vitamin K antagonist such as warfarin interferes with the synthesis of coagulation factors II, VII, IX and X by the liver. It has the great advantage of being absorbed from the alimentary tract, but with a plasma half-life of 36 hours, it does take 3–4 days to achieve a therapeutic anticoagulation level. As it has been shown that a loading dose results in an imbalance in the reduction of vitamin K dependent coagulation factors, a constant dose between 5–10 mg daily is recommended until a prothrombin time of 2–2.2 times normal is reached 3–4 days after starting treatment. The main disadvantages of warfarin therapy are the need to give doses approaching the toxic levels in order to achieve a therapeutic result, and that there is a prolonged depression in clotting factor concentration after stopping the drug.

Duration of anticoagulant therapy
For how long anticoagulant therapy should be continued following a deep vein thrombosis remains controversial. Most authorities would recommend 3 months of treatment after resolution of an acute thromboembolic episode. During this period, patients should wear elastic stockings and avoid stasis in the legs.

Contraindications to anticoagulant therapy
Anticoagulant therapy is contraindicated in hypertensives with a diastolic blood pressure greater than 110 mm Hg, in

patients with intracranial or visceral injury, in those with plate-let disorders or clotting factor deficiencies, following recent central nervous system or eye surgery, and in those with bleed-ing varices or other gastrointestinal, pulmonary or genitourinary bleeding. Oral anticoagulants are prescribed with great caution to patients with severe renal or hepatic disease or suffering from malabsorption.

Complications of anticoagulant therapy

Bleeding

Long-term anticoagulant therapy is associated with bleeding in 7–10% of patients. Should the bleeding be such as to necessitate discontinuing the anticoagulant therapy, a heparin infusion may be stopped, and a protamine titration test performed so that an accurate amount of protamine sulphate is administered. The effect of warfarin is neutralized by administering 25 mg i.v. vitamin K_1, followed by an intravenous infusion of fresh frozen plasma should bleeding continue.

Protamine sulphate

Fresh frozen plasma

A small percentage of patients (0.6%) receiving heparin develop a progressive thrombocytopenia after 6–8 days, which resolves on stopping the heparin. Long-term heparin therapy (over 6 months) may be associated with alopecia, osteoporosis and the occurrence of pathological fractures. Oral anticoag-ulant therapy is occasionally complicated by alopecia, urticaria, dermatitis, fever, nausea, diarrhoea, abdominal cramps and dermal gangrene of the thigh, breast and buttock.

Thrombocyto-penia

Iliofemoral venous thrombosis

Streptokinase

In patients with iliofemoral venous thrombosis of less than 48 hours' duration, thrombolytic therapy with streptokinase should be considered. For this to be effective, any heparin in-fusion must be stopped. Anaphylactic reactions are prevented by giving 25 mg prednisolone intravenously before a loading dose of 600 000 international units (iu) of streptokinase is administered, followed for 72 hours by an infusion at the rate of 100 000 iu per hour. On completion of this course, intravenous heparin is recommenced to prevent re-thrombosis.

Recurrent DVT

Following a deep vein thrombosis, a number of patients have repeated attacks of pain, swelling and inflammation in the leg.

Venous thromboembolism

These symptoms are usually assumed to be due to reoccurrence of the deep vein thrombosis for which a further course of anti-coagulants is prescribed. The symptoms, however, are often non-specific and may be part of the post-thrombotic syndrome rather than due to recurrent venous thrombosis.

Investigation of these patients involves Doppler studies of the deep veins, ascending venography and ^{125}I fibrinogen scanning. A normal Doppler study and venogram rule out recurrent deep venous thrombosis and some other cause of the symptoms must be found. If either the Doppler study or the venogram reveal an abnormality of the deep veins, the presence of an active thrombotic process should be sought during an attack by ^{125}I fibrinogen scanning. If this fails to show any evidence of active thrombosis, the patient can be diagnosed as suffering from the post-thrombotic syndrome and managed accordingly (Chapter 17). An abnormal ^{125}I fibrinogen uptake indicating active thrombosis is treated by anticoagulant therapy and the patient further investigated for any haematological abnormality that may predispose to a coagulopathy.

Pulmonary embolism

Clinical features

Pulmonary embolism may occur with or without the signs of a preceding deep vein thrombosis and its manifestations are non-specific and notorious for their similarity to other cardio-respiratory disorders. The diagnosis is suspected following the sudden onset of pleuritic pain associated with tachypnoea, haemoptysis and fever. There may be an associated pleural rub, localized crepitations and a pleural effusion. More major pulmonary emboli present as severe chest pain and circulatory collapse. Segmental opacities may be seen on a chest X-ray indicating areas of pulmonary infarction. Depending on the size of the embolus there will be changes in the blood gas measurements.

Pleuritic pain
Tachypnoea
Haemoptysis
Fever

Diagnosis

Pulmonary thromboembolism can be classified using simple clinical criteria and the measurement of blood gas levels. An embolus occluding less than 20% of the pulmonary artery outflow will cause no significant symptoms or signs. Occlusion of

99

Problems in peripheral vascular disease

20–30% of pulmonary artery outflow causes anxiety and hyper-ventilation with a tachycardia. Both arterial Po_2 and Pco_2 are re-duced. Collapse with dyspnoea occurs when 30–50% of the pulmonary artery outflow is occluded, the central venous pressure rises and there is further interference with gaseous ex-change and lowering of the arterial Po_2. More than 50% occlusion results in a shocked, dyspnoeic patient with a raised central venous pressure and a systemic arterial blood pressure below 100 mmHg.

Investigation

Chest X-ray
ECG
Blood gases
Lung scan

Investigations include a chest X-ray, ECG and arterial blood gas estimations. Isotopic pulmonary ventilation/perfusion scans are an accurate method of detecting pulmonary emboli provided there is no pre-existing lung disease. The most accurate method of diagnosis is achieved with the pulmonary angiogram, a tech-nique requiring catheterization of the pulmonary artery via the vena cava and the right side of the heart.

Management of pulmonary embolism

Anti-
coagulants
Thrombolytic
therapy

The majority of pulmonary emboli are managed medically with anticoagulant therapy – initially heparin infusions, followed by 3 months or so of oral anticoagulation. Thrombolytic therapy with streptokinase injected directly into the pulmonary artery via a catheter may lead to more rapid lysis of the clot with restoration of pulmonary artery perfusion and relief of right heart strain. Some pulmonary emboli are so massive that the patient dies immediately from complete occlusion of right-sided cardiac outflow. Other patients are kept alive by prompt cardio-pulmonary resuscitation and may be saved by heroic surgery in

Pulmonary
embolectomy

the form of an emergency pulmonary embolectomy with or with-out cardiopulmonary bypass. The techniques of interventional radiology now make it possible, using image intensification, to guide a trumpet-ended catheter from the femoral vein into an occluded pulmonary artery, aspirate the embolus and extract it via the venous pathway.

Recurrent pulmonary emboli

In the minority of patients who either have complications from their anticoagulant therapy, or who continue to have pulmonary emboli despite effective anticoagulation, the placement of a filter in the inferior vena cava is the present method of choice for prevention of further thromboembolic complications. Open operations to ligate, plicate or clip the superficial femoral vein or the inferior vena cava have now been superseded by transvenous placement of vena cava umbrellas which are successful in protecting patients from recurrent thromboembolism.

Vena caval umbrellas

17 The post-thrombotic syndrome

Clinical features – Venous outflow obstruction – Venous reconstructive surgery

Following damage to the deep veins of the leg associated with venous thrombosis, patients may develop a number of clinical features grouped together under the title of 'post-thrombotic syndrome'. These include stasis dermatitis, ulceration, secondary varicose veins and varying degrees of leg oedema. The two significant pathophysiological disturbances are incompetence of the deep venous valves following their destruction by the thrombotic process, and obstruction to the venous drainage of the leg by thrombus which has failed to recanalize. It is often difficult to establish clinically the relative contributions of these two abnormalities.

Clinical features

Thin legs   Patients with thin legs notice increasing venous congestions, with tense prominent veins appearing around the ankle. Sooner or later the condition of the skin begins to deteriorate with scaling and the appearance of irritating patches which the patient invariably scratches. The eczematous skin starts to weep and then becomes infected.

Fat legs   Patients with fat legs present in a different way, the subcutaneous fatty layer masking the prominent high pressure veins. The first local sign is the appearance of hard, indurated

103

areas of tissue above the medial malleolus, almost invariably diagnosed as 'phlebitis'. Untreated, the area becomes pigmented with haemosiderin due to leakage of red blood cells through the capillary walls and the skin becomes tender and inflamed, and breaks down to form an ulcer. Recent studies have shown that not only erythrocytes but also large protein molecules escape from the circulating blood into the tissues. The most important molecule is fibrinogen which polymerizes in the tissues to form an insoluble fibrin complex. This fibrin layer acts as a barrier to the exchange of nutriments and oxygen in the capillary bed resulting in cell death and ulceration. The management of these patients is described in Chapter 18.

Venous outflow obstruction

After an iliofemoral venous thrombosis (phlegmasia alba dolens, white leg) the iliac vein or inferior vena cava may be permanently narrowed or blocked. These great veins do not have any valves, so the problem is one not of valve incompetence at this level, but of interference with venous drainage from the lower limb. Unfortunately, the deep veins of the lower leg are nearly always involved in the deep venous thrombosis as well, and although these veins recanalize, their valves are no longer competent. It is this combination of venous outflow obstruction and deep vein incompetence that results in a syndrome which, although less common, is much more incapacitating and resistant to treatment.

Venous claudication Patients with venous outflow obstruction but normal valves in the lower leg suffer mainly from venous claudication. On walking any distance they develop an increasingly severe pain in the lower leg which is of a bursting nature associated with an obvious swelling and generalized congestion of the lower limb. The pain may be so severe that they have to stop walking and rest. Elevation of the leg rapidly relieves their symptoms. If there is both damage to deep vein valves and venous outflow obstruction, not only does the patient suffer from venous claudication and leg oedema, but also he or she has skin changes and ulceration.

Doppler studies The most useful non-invasive technique to assess venous problems is the Doppler ultrasound. Placing the probe over the femoral vein in the groin will allow an assessment of the patency of the iliac vein and inferior vena cava above, and the femoral vein below.

Management   A patient with venous claudication due to outflow obstruction is fitted with an elastic stocking and encouraged to exercise in order to stimulate the development of collateral venous channels. Those patients who do not improve, and whose venous claudication is particularly disabling, are investigated further by venography.

Venography   Venograms may be obtained using three main techniques. An ascending venogram is performed by injecting a radio-opaque medium into a vein on the dorsum of the foot. A tourniquet above the ankle directs the dye into the deep veins, and another below-knee tourniquet prevents it from escaping into the femoral vein until the calf veins have been visualized. Release of the tourniquet below the knee fills the femoral and iliac veins although dilution of the contrast in the large veins gives rather an indistinct radiographic appearance. Direct injection of the dye into the femoral vein itself allows better visualization of veins in the pelvis, and with the patient in a head-up position, retrograde filling of the femoral vein demonstrates valve structure and function. Contrast injected via a catheter passed through a vein in the arm down the inferior vena cava reveals abnormalities in the cava and pelvic veins.

Venous reconstructive surgery

Vein bypass   At the present time the place of direct venous surgery is controversial. Two main techniques have been applied to correct the consequences of a major ileofemoral venous thrombosis. A complete occlusion of the iliac or femoral veins can be bypassed using the patient's own long saphenous vein either by diverting venous blood to the normal venous system on the opposite side in the first case, or by simply anastomosing the distal end of the competent long saphenous vein to a calf vein in the second.

Valve grafts   Damaged valves in the region of the common femoral vein may be reconstructed by direct surgery or venous flow redirected through a segment of vein containing a competent valve by rearranging the tributaries of the common femoral vein in the groin. Transplantation of valves from the brachial vein to the femoral vein has also been attempted but is still being evaluated.

The place of venous reconstructive surgery is slowly becoming defined as the long-term results of various techniques are assessed. Bypass grafting improves venous haemodynamics and relieves patient's symptoms, but it is too early to be certain of the place of valve transplantation and most patients still require management along traditional lines.

18 Leg ulcers

Aetiology – Clinical features – Diagnosis – Management

An ulcer on the lower leg is not a disease in itself, but a manifestation of some disease process. About 1.25% of the population suffers from leg ulcer at any one time and 1–2% of all adults have, or have had, an ulcerated leg. Regrettably, the natural history of the majority of leg ulcers is influenced by the waning interest of the doctor and the gradual acceptance by the patient of a troublesome, uncomfortable, inconvenient skin lesion.

Historical aspects   The relationship between leg ulcers and varicose veins was recognized by Hippocrates, and the Romans were known to apply a variety of ointments to their ulcers and to support the limb with roller bandages. Around the time of Galen in the early centuries A.D., an ulcer was considered to be the route by which evil poisons escaped from the body, and the healing of the ulcer could be looked on as a good or bad sign depending on the circumstances! At the turn of the last century it was recognized that 'varicose' ulcers were by no means invariably associated with varicose veins, and the more accurate term 'venous' ulcer became accepted.

Aetiology

Venous insufficiency   Although 90% of leg ulcers are associated with some degree of venous insufficiency, it is important to remember that an ulcer

107

may be due to a combination of venous and arterial insufficiency in 4% of patients, and be due to ischaemia alone in another 4%. Atherosclerosis and diabetic angiopathy should be easily recognized, as should the effects of a major vascular occlusion due to arterial thrombosis or embolism. Difficulty may arise in the recognition of thromboangiitis obliterans, polyarteritis nodosa or Bazin's disease. The ulceration following cold injury or complicating chilblains can usually be diagnosed without difficulty. Congenital or acquired arteriovenous shunts may be complicated by leg ulceration. A doctor seeing a leg ulcer for the first time should bear in mind the possibility of bacterial and fungal infections, various haematological disorders and the association of leg ulcers with systemic disease. To miss a skin cancer can be particularly tragic.

Arterial insufficiency

A–V shunts

Infections

Blood disorders

Skin cancer

Diagnosis

Although the possibility of misdiagnosing a leg ulcer does exist, a venous ulcer is always associated with an 'ankle flare', a cluster of dilated venules spreading from the lower part of the ulcer across the medial malleolus to pass deep to the heel pad.

'Ankle flare'

John Homans of Boston was one of the first doctors to recognize that many venous ulcers result from a previous deep vein thrombosis. Subsequent studies have confirmed this observation, and by use of ascending venography to investigate patients with venous ulcers, 80–90% have been shown to have some abnormality in the venous drainage of the lower limb attributable to deep vein thrombosis. Many patients, however, are unable to give a convincing history of such an event. Primary varicose veins are not usually the basic cause of leg ulcers, although up to a quarter of patients with leg ulcers have neglected varicosities. The majority of venous ulcers are a feature of the post-thrombotic syndrome, the actual onset of ulceration being precipitated by an episode of minor trauma to the skin.

Deep vein abnormalities

Post-thrombotic syndrome

Clinical features

Venous ulcers are found above the ankle joint in the gaiter area of the lower limb. The skin and subcutaneous tissue is oedematous and thickened, with a surrounding zone of varying degrees of inflammation and pigmentation. Venous ulcers may be single or multiple; medial, lateral or circumferential; in shape, oval or serpiginous. The edge of such an ulcer is always

Ulcer

Overtreatment

flat and sloping. Any suggestion of a punched-out ulcer or eversion of the edge raises the suspicion of some other aetiology. The ulcer never penetrates muscle, and bone is never exposed although the periosteum may be thickened. The base of the ulcer is covered with an infected slough from which arises a purulent discharge of varying degrees of profuseness and offensiveness. Neglect by the patient or overtreatment by the doctor or nurse often results in the surrounding skin being caked with dried pus and serum lying on scales of skin, or in an extensive weeping eczema due to tissue sensitization by some topical medicament aggravated by maceration from the purulent discharge and an occlusive dressing.

Management

History

The history will include details of the mode of onset and duration of the ulceration, and whether the ulcer has ever healed before breaking down again and if so under what circumstances. Details of any medical or surgical treatment for varicose veins is noted, and the patient questioned about the possibility of a previous deep vein thrombosis or episode of thrombophlebitis. Particular care is taken to identify patients with peripheral vascular disease, or those who have had a course of radiotherapy to the ulcerated area in the past. A note is made of the patient's general health, past medical history and any specific drug therapy, with attention being paid to any condition that may be associated with leg oedema.

Examination

Examination of the patient, following a rapid appraisal of general habits, socio-economic group and level of intelligence, is usually confined to the lower limbs. The site, size and appearance of the ulcerated area are recorded, together with the state of the surrounding skin. Varicosities of the long and short saphenous veins are sought, and the sites of possible incompetent perforating veins identified. The presence of palpable ankle pulses usually excludes significant arterial disease.

Investigation

Swabs are usually taken for bacteriological examination when the patient first presents, although in the absence of a widespread cellulitis no systemic antibiotic treatment is required. Any suspicious ulcer, or one that has been present for over 12 months, should be biopsied. Wedges of tissue are removed from each of the four quadrants after infiltration with a local anaesthetic. Investigation of the post-thrombotic syndrome has been discussed in Chapter 17.

Medical management

As venous ulcers are caused by local venous hypertension, all these ulcers can be cured by one of three modes of treatment: (1) elevate the feet above the level of the heart, (2) apply an equal and opposite pressure to that exerted in the ulcer and surrounding tissues and (3) correct the abnormal mechanism causing venous hypertension.

Elevate feet   All venous ulcers will heal if the patient is treated by bed rest with the feet elevated so that the ulcer is above the level of the heart. This is seldom practicable, prolonged bed rest having its own complications particularly in the elderly. Moreover, the ulcer reoccurs soon after the patient resumes a vertical posture. However, a short period of complete bed rest with high elevation of the feet is often the only way to start reversing the deleterious effects of venous hypertension in the longstanding, neglected ulcer.

Contact dermatitis and eczema   All too often these patients have developed local skin sensitization to various topical applications, and have an area of inflamed, eczematous skin around the ulcer. Many antibiotic creams and ointments have been incriminated, together with lanolin, preservative agents found in most proprietary topical agents, local anaesthetic and antihistamine creams and even rubber additives in the elasticated bandages and stockings. Occasionally the hypersensitivity becomes generalized – the patient presenting with itching eczematous lesions on the lower limbs, forearms and trunk. Once any potential allergen has been withdrawn, gross sepsis controlled, the ulcer cleaned and the surrounding skin descaled, a 24–48 h application of topical steroid (either hydrocortisone cream or steroid-impregnated cotton bandage) will bring relief of symptoms and resolution of the dermatitis. Patients troubled by a generalized eczema usually respond to a short course of systemic steroids (prednisolone 5 mg thrice daily for 5 days).

General measures   Nearly all patients with chronic venous ulcers have some

110

treatable reversible disease. The oedema of cardiac failure or hypoproteinaemia should be corrected, obese patients encouraged to lose weight and diabetics identified and treated.

Local treatment
The aim of local treatment is to control infection and the adjacent dermatitis. Scales and crusts are removed from the edge of the ulcer with dissecting forceps and the ulcer cleaned with either normal saline or half-strength eusol solution. Occasionally desloughing agents are required in the early days of management. There is no particular advantage in applying reconstituted freeze-dried pig skin, human amnion or a variety of other organic and inorganic dressings. Although antiseptics destroy pathogenic organisms, they also cause some degree of tissue necrosis and delay healing. Antibiotics should be reserved for the treatment of a widespread cellulitis.

Outpatient care
Once sepsis and dermatitis have responded to active treatment, the patient may be treated as an outpatient. After the ulcer has been cleaned, it is covered with dry gauze over which is placed either a 13 mm (half-inch) thick rubber or plastic sponge, or an equal layer of absorbent gamgee. Subcutaneous venous hypertension is controlled by the application of an elasticated bandage from toes to below knee. In the initial stages of ambulatory management, the ulcer may need to be dressed two or three times a week, but once there are clean, pink granulations over which an iris or bluish epithelium is creeping, the ulcer is dressed at increasingly longer intervals. When discharge is minimal, the application of an aqueous solution of gentian violet 2% will help to dry up the ulcer, the gentian violet having mild antiseptic properties. During this latter phase of the healing process, scales of dry skin are gently removed at every opportunity, as it is the growth of bacteria under this desquamated epidermis which can lead to the reappearance of infection with an increasing purulent discharge and surrounding dermatitis.

Treating the cause
Once the ulcer has healed, further management is always necessary to prevent reoccurrence. Venograms nearly always reveal evidence of previous extensive damage to the deep veins and may confirm the presence of incompetent perforators 'feeding' the ulcer. A course of compression sclerotherapy aimed at sealing these perforators is a logical step in preventing recurrence and 89% cure rates at 4–5 years have been claimed for this approach. On the other hand, the surgical approach with ligation of the perforators, usually in the subfascial position, has been associated with the recurrence of the ulcer in 50% of patients despite encouraging early results.

111

Surgical management

Surgery for venous ulcers should be directed towards (1) dealing with any gross varicosities, (2) ligation of incompetent perforating veins and (3) excision of a chronic persisting or recurrent ulcer. Any venous ulcer that has been present for over a year is unlikely to heal satisfactorily. Even if it does epithelialize with the help of enthusiastic conservative measures, the skin cover is so thin that it soon breaks down again. These ulcers need to be excised and grafted. Usually this requires a period of inpatient care for assessment of the patient generally, and the active management of what is usually a neglected and infected ulcer. The aim of surgery is to excise the ulcer with a wide margin together with its fibrous tissue floor down to, and often including, the deep fascia and sometimes even the periosteum. This excision can often be combined with a subfascial ligation of perforating veins. It is usually inadvisable to carry out a partial thickness skin graft at the same time; it is preferable to take and store the graft in saline solution in a refrigerator at $-4\,°C$ for 7–10 days. By then the excised ulcer will be granulating, the grafting is carried out and the skin graft can be kept in position by firm bandaging for another week or so. The inpatient management of these ulcers may necessitate a stay in hospital of 4–6 weeks.

The education of the patient in the pathogenesis and management of his or her ulcer has a great influence on the success of all methods of treatment. Results of treating venous ulcers in private practice are often better than in the general population. This is partly due to the interest shown by the doctor, but is also associated with the interest shown by the patient!

Even when an ulcer has healed, continuing care is required to prevent recurrence. Any tendency towards obesity or leg oedema must be corrected. The wearing of thick stockings or even shinpads helps to avoid episodes of minor trauma to the lower leg which so often lead to skin breakdown. Daily elevation of the legs reduces oedema, the most effective method being to lie flat with the legs resting vertically up a wall. Elastic stockings should be made to measure and replaced before they lose all their elasticity, and be worn whenever the patient is in a vertical position.

Ligate perforators

Excision and grafting

Education

Prophylaxis

Index